CRAIG THURMOND

The Garden Guide "Fun facts for Budding Green Thumb's"

Fun Facts for Budding Green Thumbs

Copyright © 2025 by Craig Thurmond

All rights reserved. No part of this publication may be reproduced, stored or transmitted in any form or by any means, electronic, mechanical, photocopying, recording, scanning, or otherwise without written permission from the publisher. It is illegal to copy this book, post it to a website, or distribute it by any other means without permission.

First edition

This book was professionally typeset on Reedsy. Find out more at reedsy.com

This book is dedicated to all of my family and clients over the last 35 years. Thanks for allowing me to work with you and learn from my experiences.

Contents

Introduction	1
Chapter 1	5
Starting Your Green Adventure	6
Chapter 2	25
Fun Facts and Fascinating Flora	25
Chapter 3	45
Interactive Gardening Adventures	46
Chapter 4	68
Sustainable Gardening Practices	69
Chapter 5	88
Garden as Art	88
Chapter 6	109
Problem-Solving and Practical Tip	109
Chapter 7	127
Gardening with Community and Connection	128
Chapter 8	165
Conclusion	165
Chapter 9	170
References	170

Introduction

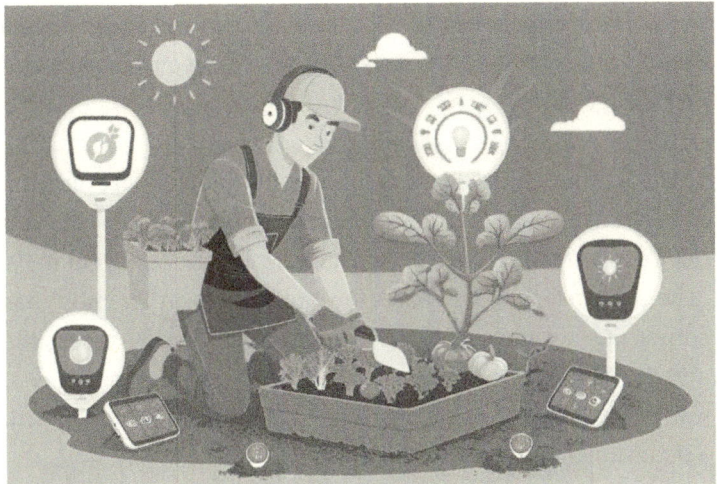

Let me share a little secret that every gardener learns sooner or later: plants are just as quirky as people. Some like the sun, others thrive in the shade. Some are always thirsty, while others are more like camels, needing water only now and then. It's these quirks that make gardening such an intriguing adventure. Imagine planting a seed and watching it sprout, grow, and bloom, each stage full of surprises. It's a dance with nature, one that never gets old.

THE GARDEN GUIDE "FUN FACTS FOR BUDDING GREEN THUMB'S"

I'm Craig R. Thurmond, and I've been working with gardens for over 35 years. I graduated from the University of Georgia with a degree in landscape architecture back in 1990 and taught Horticulture for about ten years at North Georgia Technical College. Since then, I've rolled up my sleeves and dug into the dirt, literally and figuratively. My journey has taken me through countless gardens worldwide in my professional work and at home in North Georgia, where I live with my family. My wife and two kids have seen me marvel at tiny sprouts and cheer when a design comes to life. Now, I want to share that enthusiasm and knowledge with you.

This book is a guide, a companion, and a source of inspiration for anyone looking to dig into gardening. Whether you're a novice just starting out or an old hand with soil under your nails, "The Garden Guide: Fun Facts for Budding Green Thumbs" has something for you. My goal is to make gardening accessible and enjoyable for everyone, regardless of age or experience. I want to help you grow your garden IQ from the ground up, with a bit of fun along the way.

In these pages, you'll find more than just instructions on how to plant tomatoes or cultivate roses. You'll discover practical tips and engaging projects that can transform your backyard into a thriving oasis. Whether you're interested in growing your own vegetables, creating stunning flower beds, or designing a landscape that wows, this book has you covered. And let's not forget the joy of gardening as a family activity. There's nothing quite like seeing a child's eyes light up when they pick the first ripe strawberry they helped grow.

INTRODUCTION

Who is this book for? Well, it's for anyone with a curiosity about growing things. Whether you're an adult looking to landscape your yard, a gardener aiming to expand your knowledge, or simply someone with a budding interest in plants, you'll find valuable insights here. Landscapers, hobbyists, and even those who think they have a "black thumb" will find this book a helpful friend on their gardening journey.

Here's a sneak peek of what's inside. You'll find fun facts about plants that will make great conversation starters. There are hands-on projects that are as entertaining as they are educational. You'll learn about sustainable practices that benefit your garden and the planet. I've also included creative ideas that will inspire you to try new things and see your garden in a new light.

Expect an interactive experience. This book is more than just words on a page. It's an invitation to get your hands dirty. Think of it as your personal gardening toolkit, filled with ideas and inspiration. I hope to spark your curiosity and encourage you to explore, try, and learn. Gardening is a lifelong journey, one that offers endless opportunities for discovery. It connects us to the earth and each other, fostering a deeper appreciation for nature and all it provides.

As you turn the pages, I invite you to dig into the wealth of knowledge and creativity that awaits you. Let this book be your guide on a rewarding gardening adventure. Together, we'll explore the wonders of the plant world and find joy in watching things grow. So, grab your gardening gloves, and let's get started!

THE GARDEN GUIDE "FUN FACTS FOR BUDDING GREEN THUMB'S"

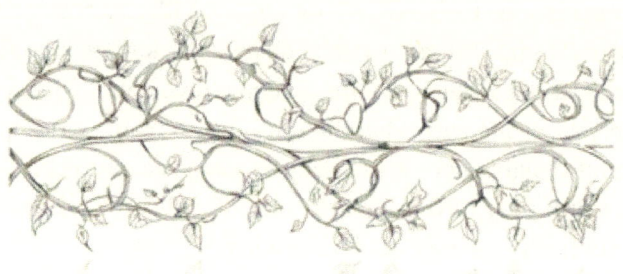

Chapter 1

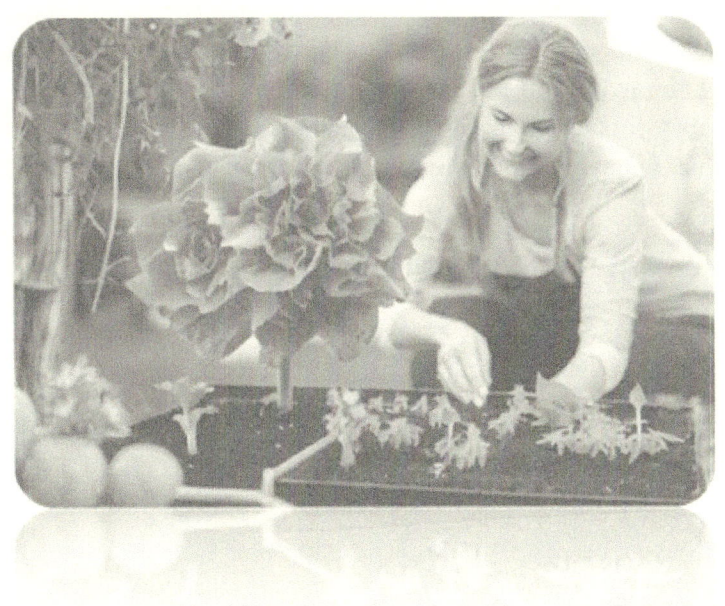

THE GARDEN GUIDE "FUN FACTS FOR BUDDING GREEN THUMB'S"

Starting Your Green Adventure

Did you know that the oldest known plant lineage still gracing our planet today dates back millions of years? That's right, mosses and their relatives have been hanging around since before dinosaurs roamed the earth. Imagine what gardening secrets they might whisper if only we could understand their ancient language. This fascinating tidbit is just a taste of the wonders you'll encounter as you start your green adventure. Whether you're here to cultivate a relaxing hobby, beautify your backyard, or grow your own fresh produce, this chapter is your gateway. We will explore some of the quirkiest, most captivating plant facts that will expand your gardening knowledge and make you the star of any garden party conversation.

CHAPTER 1

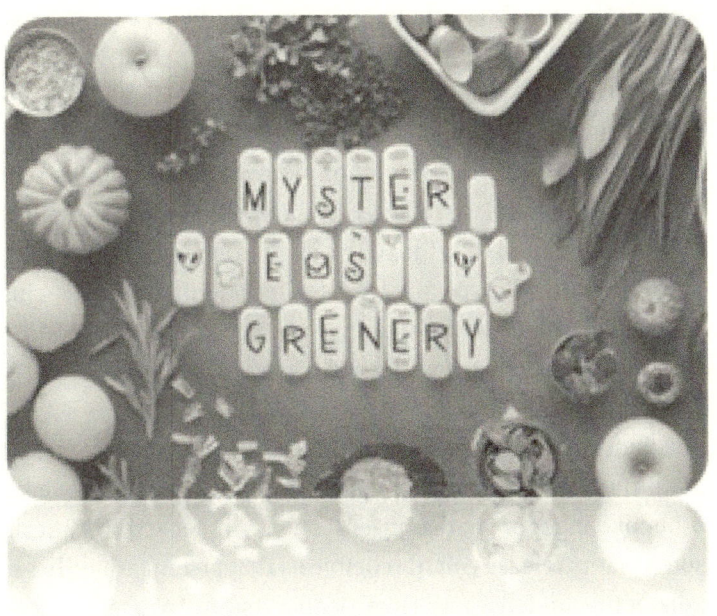

Unveiling Plant Mysteries: Fun Facts to Get You Hooked

Let's kick things off with the carnivorous plants. You read that right: some plants have adopted a predatory lifestyle! Take the Venus flytrap, for instance. This little marvel has specialized leaves that snap shut when unsuspecting insects wander too close. It's not just a freak show; it's an adaptation to nutrient-poor soils where these plants thrive by drawing nutrients from their prey. And they're not alone. Pitcher plants lure insects into their deep, slippery wells, where escape becomes impossible. It's like a botanical roller coaster with no return ticket.

THE GARDEN GUIDE "FUN FACTS FOR BUDDING GREEN THUMB'S"

Now, let's talk about plants that literally dance to their own tune. The Mimosa pudica, often called the "sensitive plant," is famous for its dramatic reaction to touch. Give it a gentle nudge, and its leaves fold up faster than you can say "photosynthesis." This phenomenon, known as thigmonasty, is a defense mechanism to deter herbivores. Meanwhile, some plants are reputed to respond to music. Sound waves influence plant growth, with specific frequencies potentially enhancing their yield. Imagine serenading your tomatoes with a bit of classical music and watching them grow in response!

Speaking of plant conversations, did you know that plants can communicate? Through chemical signaling, they warn each other of danger or share nutrients. When under attack by pests, some plants release volatile chemicals that alert nearby allies to bolster their defenses. It's like a leafy version of a neighborhood watch program. Fascinatingly, certain studies have shown that plants can even respond to sound vibrations, such as the gentle hum of flowing water, guiding roots toward moisture sources.

Nature's adaptability doesn't stop there. Consider desert flora like cacti and succulents, which have mastered water conservation through thickened leaves and specialized storage tissues. These adaptations ensure survival in harsh environments where rain is as rare as a snowstorm in the Sahara. Meanwhile, alpine plants have evolved to withstand extreme cold by growing low to the ground and producing antifreeze proteins.

Let's not forget about edible plants with unexpected benefits. Microgreens, tiny seedlings of edible vegetables and herbs, are packed with nutrients, often boasting higher vitamin content than their mature counterparts. These little powerhouses are not just garnish; they're superfoods in disguise! And then, there are herbs like basil and rosemary, which add flavor to your dishes and contain compounds with potential medicinal properties. From boosting immunity to improving digestion, they truly are nature's pharmacy.

As you embark on this botanical adventure, you'll discover that there's more to plants than meets the eye. They're not just passive greenery; they're dynamic organisms with stories to tell and secrets to share. Whether it's through adapting to extreme environments, communicating with their kin, or offering health benefits, plants are endlessly fascinating. So grab your gardening gloves and get ready to uncover the mysteries hidden in your backyard!

THE GARDEN GUIDE "FUN FACTS FOR BUDDING GREEN THUMB'S"

Green Thumbs 101: Building Confidence in Your Gardening Abilities

Starting a garden can feel like walking into a room where everyone speaks a different language. But fear not because growing plants don't require translating ancient hieroglyphics.

CHAPTER 1

Let's begin with the basics. Choosing the right soil is crucial. Think of soil as the bed your plants sleep in; too hard and they won't rest; too soft and they'll sink. You want a Goldilocks situation—just right. A good rule of thumb is to look for well-draining soil that retains moisture without drowning your plants. Containers matter, too. They're like the shoes of the plant world. Too tight, and roots get cramped; too loose, and they flop about. Opt for containers with drainage holes to prevent waterlogged roots.

Next, pick your plant pals wisely. Start simple with hardy, easy-to-grow varieties like marigolds or radishes. These reliable friends won't ghost you after a week. They're forgiving and thrive with minimal fuss. Whether you have a sprawling backyard or a cozy balcony, these plants won't disappoint you.

Once you're set-up, it's all about nurturing. Watering is both an art and a science. Too much water, and you risk drowning your seedlings; too little, and they'll look at you with wilted disappointment. Aim for a consistent schedule to minimize evaporation, ideally early in the morning or late afternoon. A good soak every few days is better than daily sprinkles.

Plants are like toddlers; they sometimes throw tantrums for no apparent reason. Recognizing common ailments is part of the fun. Yellowing leaves might mean your plant needs more nitrogen, while droopy stems could signal overwatering. Keep an eye out for pests, too. A quick once-over daily can save you from future headaches.

Now, let's talk about the tools of the trade. You don't need to invest in a shed full of gadgets to start gardening. Focus on the essentials that make life easier. A hand trowel is invaluable for digging small holes and transplanting. Pruners help manage growth and remove dead bits. They're like your garden's haircut scissors, snip snip! And don't underestimate the power of good gloves. They protect against thorns and keep your hands dirt-free, though some might say dirt is just a gardener's badge of honor.

Gardening involves plenty of bending and kneeling, which can be hard on the knees. Enter kneeling pads—a gardener's best friend for comfort. They cushion you from the hard ground, making long planting sessions more bearable.

Gardening isn't about getting it perfect right away. It's about learning as you grow, pun intended! Embrace the trial-and-error process. It's okay if a plant doesn't thrive; it's all part of nature's learning curve. Celebrate small victories, like the first bloom or sprout. These milestones are what make gardening so rewarding.

A growth mindset is key here. Skills develop over time with practice and patience. Don't get discouraged by initial setbacks or challenges. Each season brings new opportunities to try again and improve.

Gardening Confidence Checklist

- Choose well-draining soil
- Select easy-to-grow plants
- Water consistently in the early mornings

CHAPTER 1

- Use essential tools: hand trowel, pruners, gloves
- Embrace trial and error
- Celebrate every small success

Approach gardening with curiosity and wonder, not as a chore but as an adventure in green-thumb development. Every gardener started somewhere, usually with an overwatered cactus or a pot of parsley that refused to sprout. The beauty lies in keeping at it and watching how each plant teaches you something new about patience, resilience, and life.

Remember, gardening isn't just about plants; it's about growth in every sense of the word. As you work with soil and seeds, you also nurture your understanding and capabilities. It's a dance with nature that becomes more graceful with every step you take. So, grab those gloves, pick up your trowel, and confidently jump into your garden!

Garden Mythbusters: Debunking Common Gardening Misconceptions

Gardening myths are like persistent weeds in the fertile soil of our minds; once planted, they can spread rapidly. Let's tackle one of the most tenacious myths out there: the notion that a "green thumb" is necessary for successful gardening. I promise you, no magical appendage is required to nurture plants. Instead, you need a willingness to learn and a bit of patience. Imagine if everyone believed that only naturally athletic people could play sports; we'd have empty fields and courts. Similarly, gardening is a skill anyone can cultivate through practice and curiosity, not some innate talent exclusive to a select few.

Another oft-repeated myth is that all plants crave full sun. While it's true that some species bask in the sunlight like sunbathers on a Florida beach, others are more like vampires, preferring the cool embrace of shade. Shade-loving plants like ferns and hostas thrive in indirect light, turning shady corners into lush retreats. Understanding this can save you from the heartbreak of watching sun-sensitive plants wither under intense rays. The key lies in knowing your plants' preferences and adapting your garden to suit them, like tailoring a wardrobe to fit your lifestyle.

Let's use some science to investigate these misconceptions. Plants don't just rely on sunlight; they depend on soil health, too. Imagine soil as your plants' pantry, stocked with the nutrients they need to grow strong. While genetics plays a role, soil quality often determines success. Quality soil acts as both a support system and a nutrient reservoir. By maintaining rich, well-aerated soil, you significantly boost your garden's potential, turning even the most stubborn patches into fertile ground.

Please question gardening advice and seek out reliable sources. Not all gardening wisdom is created equal; some tips get passed down like old wives' tales without scientific backing. Find information on reputable gardening websites or university extensions that provide research-based insights. Cross-referencing multiple sources can help confirm facts and dispel myths. It's like an investigator piecing together a botanical puzzle, where every confirmed fact clarifies your gardening

CHAPTER 1

picture.

Debunking these myths can transform your gardening experience. When you let go of the pressure to have a green thumb, you open the door to experimentation and enjoyment. You might find yourself trying new plants or techniques without fear of failure. Understanding the range of light conditions plants thrive in allows you to design more diverse gardens with healthier plants. It's like discovering that you've been playing with only half the pieces of a chess set—suddenly, you have more strategies at your disposal.

Take this newfound freedom and run with it! Experiment with different plant placements based on their light needs or test new soil amendments to improve fertility. As your confidence grows, so too will your willingness to try innovative ideas, leading to gardens that reflect your unique vision and personality. By breaking free of these misconceptions, you'll see improvements in plant health and yield and enjoy the process more. Gardening becomes less about getting everything right, and more about celebrating the quirks and surprises nature throws your way.

The impact of busting these myths extends beyond just better gardening results; it enhances your overall enjoyment of the hobby. When false beliefs do not bog you down, you're free to explore, experiment, and engage with your garden in new and exciting ways. This openness leads to more rewarding experiences and a deeper connection with the natural world around you. As you continue on this path, you'll find that each season brings fresh opportunities for learning and growth, enriching your garden and life.

Kid-Friendly Gardens: Creating a Magical Green Space for Children

Imagine, if you will, a garden transformed into a veritable wonderland for children, where every leaf, every petal seems to whisper secrets, and every hidden nook beckons with endless possibilities. Designing such a space requires mastering a delicate balance between safety and the wondrous enchantment that captures a child's imagination. Begin your garden adventure with raised beds, carefully crafted and placed within easy reach for those small, eager hands. These elevated plots offer more than just protection for your precious plants from trampling feet; they serve as welcoming platforms, inviting children to immerse themselves fully in the joys of gardening. By choosing non-toxic, pet-friendly blooms such as the towering sunflowers, the cheery marigolds, and the enchanting snapdragons, you infuse the garden with vibrant hues while ensuring there's no risk to the young explorers. With these thoughtful choices, you transform your garden into a sanctuary, a safe haven where children can roam and discover the wonders of nature without a hint of worry.

Hands-On Activities: Bringing the Garden to Life

Incorporating hands-on activities into this green space turns gardening from a mere passive experience into an exhilarating adventure. Fast-growing seeds like radishes and those with almost magical properties in their growth speed captivate young minds with their incredible transformation from tiny seeds to edible delight. Encourage kids to plant these seeds with anticipation, water them lovingly, and witness the miracle unfold before their eyes. Creating a simple yet fascinating worm compost bin also provides another interactive project that delights children. Worms, those wriggling little creatures, hold a special allure for kids, and this activity subtly introduces them to the concept of recycling organic waste into nutrient-rich soil. It becomes an eco-friendly lesson in sustainability, cleverly disguised as play. The thrill of seeing worms at work turning scraps into soil—transforms what could easily become mundane into a captivating, engaging science experiment that they will talk about for weeks.

Cultivating Wonder and Responsibility

Fostering a sense of wonder and responsibility in children is essential in nurturing a deep and lasting connection with nature. Employ time-lapse photography to capture the invisible-to-the-eye magic of plant growth, an unfolding of life from the first diminutive sprout to a fully grown, flourishing flower or vegetable. Watching these sped-up transformations nurtures patience and curiosity within their young minds, like having a coveted front-row seat to nature's most spectacular theatre. Encourage the little gardeners to maintain a garden journal, an indispensable tool where they can draw colorful pictures or scribble down their observations and experiments. This simple activity enhances literacy skills and serves as a precious, personal record of their adventurous journey in gardening.

An Educational Bounty

The educational aspects of gardening are both vast and varied, offering profound lessons across a multitude of subjects. Introduce the basics of biology by exploring the intricate stages of the plant life cycle and delve into the mysteries of photosynthesis. Explain how plants harness sunlight to make food, cleverly drawing parallels to how we consume food to fuel our bodies. Gardening also offers natural lessons in ecology, demonstrating the intricate interactions between plants, animals, and insects within an ecosystem. Math skills indirectly come into play as children enthusiastically measure plant growth or joyfully count leaves and petals. Through these simple yet effective activities, your garden morphs into an outdoor classroom where learning unfolds seamlessly and effortlessly.

To create this magical green space, start on a small scale and build gradually, keeping momentum while preserving enthusiasm. Whether a modest corner of your garden or a sunny balcony, any space can evolve into a realm of discovery and growth for your children. As they actively engage and interact with the garden, immersing themselves in the greenness, they learn about plants and responsibility, care, and commitment. Watching over their little patch of earth instills a burgeoning sense of pride and ownership that eventually extends beyond the garden into other areas of life.

So gather those gardening gloves for yourself and the eager youngsters and start sowing seeds for future memories that will last a lifetime. Transform your garden into a place where curiosity blossoms alongside vibrant flowers, where every visit is a journey filled with discovery and delight. In this unique and special space, your children will grow plants and cultivate an enduring love and respect for nature and learning. Here, in the gentle, nurturing embrace of the garden, they'll find more than

CHAPTER 1

just greenery but an opportunity for personal growth, becoming budding stewards of the earth in their own small but significant way.

Gardening for the Space-Challenged: Maximizing Small Areas

Gardening in tight spaces can seem daunting, but with a bit of creativity, even the smallest area can burst with life. Vertical gardening techniques are a fantastic way to maximize limited space. By thinking upwards rather than outwards, you can transform bare walls or fences into lush, living canvases. Trellises or wall-mounted planters are key tools in this endeavor. Imagine a cascade of climbing beans or peas reaching skywards, their tendrils gripping support structures like acrobats on a trapeze. These climbers save ground space and add a vertical element to your garden that draws the eye and adds dimension.

Container gardening is another strategy for maximizing small areas. This approach lets you turn everyday household items into unique planters. An old colander, with its built-in drainage holes, becomes a quirky herb garden. A vintage suitcase lined with plastic offers a charming home for succulents. The possibilities are as limitless as your imagination. When selecting plants for containers, opt for compact or dwarf varieties. These petite versions of their full-sized counterparts thrive in confined spaces, making them ideal for patios, balconies, or even windowsills.

Indoor gardening presents yet another opportunity for those space-challenged gardeners. Your home's interior can become a thriving ecosystem with minimal space and effort. Window sills and shelves make perfect platforms for an indoor garden. Picture a row of small pots filled with fragrant herbs like basil or mint, ready to be snipped and added to your next culinary masterpiece. Microgreens, tiny yet packed with nutrients, grow happily indoors, requiring only a shallow dish and a sliver of sunlight to flourish. Their quick growth cycle and vibrant colors make them a rewarding choice for novice gardeners.

Maximize your available light and resources to ensure your plants thrive indoors or in small outdoor spaces. Reflective materials, like mirrors or white surfaces, can amplify natural light, creating a brighter environment for your plants to soak up the sun's rays. It's like giving your garden a built-in spotlight! Efficient watering systems are also crucial in small gardens where overwatering can quickly lead to soggy soil and unhappy plants. Drip irrigation systems or self-watering pots ensure that your plants receive just the right amount of moisture without waste.

Consider the story of Clara, who transformed her tiny apartment balcony into a verdant paradise using these techniques. With limited space and no ground to plant, she turned to vertical gardening, installing narrow wooden trellises along the balcony railings. She trained her peas to climb these structures while her strawberries cascaded beautifully from wall-mounted planters above. By repurposing colorful tin cans as herb planters and clustering them on sunny windowsills inside her home, she created a seamless blend of indoor and outdoor spaces lush with greenery.

CHAPTER 1

Clara's success lies in her ability to think creatively about her space limitations. She leveraged vertical surfaces, unconventional containers, and careful plant selection to cultivate a thriving garden that defied its physical constraints. Her story illustrates how even the most cramped quarters can yield bountiful results with some ingenuity and effort.

For those worried about space, remember that a garden's size doesn't determine its impact or beauty. Even a single pot on a windowsill can bring joy and satisfaction. Gardening is about nurturing life and finding peace in the process, whether in a sprawling field or a square foot of earth.

Some might argue that smaller gardens offer unique advantages over larger ones. They require less work overall, allowing for more intimate interactions with each plant. You can observe changes daily and make adjustments swiftly. Plus, the challenges of working within constraints often lead to more innovative solutions and greater personal satisfaction when things flourish.

So, embrace your small space! Approach it as an opportunity for creativity rather than a limitation. With vertical gardens reaching the sky and colorful containers dotting every available surface, your little patch of earth can become an oasis of greenery that rivals any more extensive garden in beauty and productivity.

Seasonal Gardening: Your Year-Round Guide to Thriving Plants

As the seasons shift, so too should your gardening strategies. Think of your garden as a bustling stage, with different plants taking the spotlight as the year progresses. Cool-season crops like spinach, kale, and broccoli love the brisk chill of early spring or fall, thriving when the air is crisp and the sun is less intense. These resilient greens are the first to brave the garden in spring and the last to linger as winter approaches. On the other hand, warm-season crops are the heat-seekers of the plant world. Tomatoes, peppers, and cucumbers revel in the summer sun, growing vigorously when temperatures soar. Timing is crucial; plant them after the last frost to ensure they flourish in the long, warm days ahead.

Bulbs and tubers have their own rhythm, requiring a bit of foresight. Tulips and daffodils need a cold spell to ignite their springtime glory, so plant them in the fall when the earth begins its cool descent. This chilling period spurs their development, ensuring a vibrant display when spring arrives. Meanwhile, summer-blooming bulbs like dahlias and lilies prefer a spring start, soaking up warmth as they prepare for their late-summer grand entrance.

Seasonal challenges are part of gardening's charm and its trials. Frost can be a formidable foe for tender plants. But fear not, for there are ways to shield your garden from its icy grip. On frosty nights, cloak delicate plants with old sheets or blankets, creating a cozy barrier against the chill. For more permanent solutions, consider investing in floating row covers or frost cloths that hover over plants, offering protection without suffocating them.

CHAPTER 1

Drought conditions present another hurdle. Water becomes a precious commodity when rain is scarce. Drip irrigation systems are your best friend here, delivering moisture directly to the roots with minimal waste. Mulching is another effective strategy; a layer of organic material like straw or wood chips retains soil moisture and reduces evaporation. It's like giving your garden a protective hat against the sun's harsh rays.

Planning is a gardener's secret weapon. A seasonal gardening calendar serves as both a roadmap and a record-keeper. Jot down planting dates and tasks to stay organized and on track. Track growth patterns and harvests to learn from each season's successes and mishaps. This living document evolves with your garden, helping you refine your approach year after year.

For those of you itching for more, extending the growing season is entirely doable with a few clever techniques. Cold frames, essentially miniature greenhouses, trap heat from the sun, creating a microclimate that shields plants from cold snaps while allowing sunlight in. These structures extend your growing window, letting you harvest greens well into fall or even winter.

Greenhouses offer even greater possibilities, providing a haven where tropical plants can thrive even when snow blankets the ground outside. Think of them as your personal Eden, where you control climate and conditions to cultivate a lush paradise year-round.

Succession planting keeps your garden productive without interruption. By staggering plantings every few weeks, you ensure a continuous harvest throughout the growing season.

THE GARDEN GUIDE "FUN FACTS FOR BUDDING GREEN THUMB'S"

As soon as one crop is ready to retire, another is poised to take its place, ensuring your table remains laden with fresh produce.

Imagine a typical gardener named Sarah who embraced these strategies with gusto. Her spring garden bursts with leafy greens by April, followed by tomatoes and peppers taking center stage in July. As fall approaches, she seamlessly transitions back to cool-season crops like carrots and beets, employing cold frames to extend their life well into November. Each season brings unique challenges, but Sarah relishes them as opportunities for learning and growth.

By embracing seasonal gardening, you maximize your garden's potential and deepen your connection to nature's rhythms. Each season offers new lessons and rewards those willing to adapt and experiment. So grab your calendar, dust off those cold frames, and prepare to dance through the seasons with your plants leading the way.

As you cultivate your garden year-round, remember that it's not just about what you grow but how you grow alongside it. Through each season's trials and triumphs, you'll discover that gardening is as much about nurturing yourself as it is about nurturing plants. In tending to your plot of earth, you find yourself rooted more firmly in life's cycles, a part of something larger than any single season could encompass.

Chapter 2

Fun Facts and Fascinating Flora

Plant Superpowers: The Incredible Abilities of Everyday Flora

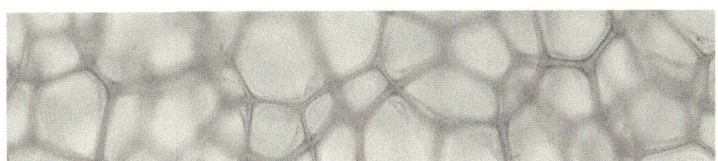

Allow me to indulge your curiosity with a captivating tidbit that will perhaps leave you astounded and may even make your garden spade seem like an accessory of magic: Did you know that certain plants possess the astonishing capacity to purify their surroundings, acting as verdant custodians of our environment? It's akin to having a chlorophyll-infused crusader right there in your backyard. This extraordinary phenomenon is facilitated by a process known as phytoremediation. With this remarkable skill, select plants can absorb detrimental contaminants through their root systems, effectively extracting and neutralizing toxins from soil and water sources. Consider sunflowers, for example, which have been utilized in environmental science to rehabilitate sites contaminated with radioactive materials. Envision an expanse of bright sunflowers lifting spirits with their sunny disposition and actively purifying the land beneath them. A testament to nature's inherent power and a marvel in its own right!

CHAPTER 2

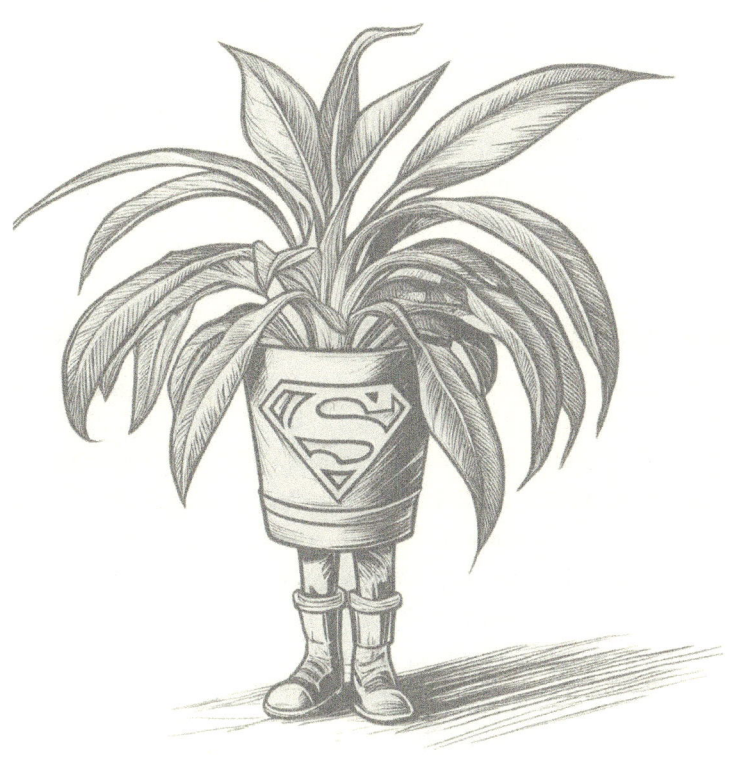

Delving deeper into these remarkable plant powers, we must shine a light on the process of photosynthesis. This might seem like an everyday miracle known to many, yet its complexity and significance remain underappreciated. Photosynthesis is the wondrous biochemical operation through which plants ingeniously transform sunlight into energy, effectively oper-

27

ating like organic solar generators. Indeed, without this vital process, our existence, as it stands, would be inconceivable. By absorbing carbon dioxide alongside the sunlight, plants synthesize oxygen and glucose. This sustains their own growth and development and all aerobic life forms by contributing the very oxygen that fills our lungs. Imagine sitting beneath the cooling shade of a sprawling tree; take a moment to acknowledge and express gratitude for the oxygen you inhale, thanks to these silent green laborers.

Yet, the prowess of plants extends far beyond any singular function; they embody nature's versatility, having adapted and evolved to surmount some of life's harshest challenges. Consider the tenacity of desert plants, nature's maestros of conservation and resilience, thriving amid relentless heat and scarce water availability. Masterpieces of design, such as cacti, epitomize this adaptive ingenuity, with their tough, waxy skin acting as a formidable barrier against evaporation. At the same time, their flesh serves as an expansive reservoir for precious moisture. They skillfully preserve moisture by employing microscopic portals termed stomata, which can seal shut during the zenith of daylight heat. Through such ingenious adaptations, they transform the unyielding desert into survivable realms, thriving where others would wither away.

In contrast, some species have mastered survival in subdued illumination, flourishing in low-light environments that might spell desolation for others. Shade-tolerant plants have fine-tuned their physiology to prosper where others struggle to exist. Take ferns and hostas, for instance, as luminaries of this adaptation, thriving under a forest canopy or in secluded garden corners. Their expansive leaf surfaces capture any fragment of light available, optimizing their photosynthetic efficiency even under the sparsest rays. It is as if these plants have mastered making much of scant resources—a lesson of frugality and resilience that humans might well imbibe with humble admiration.

Now, let's wander into the enchanting realm of plants that moonlight as healers and rejuvenators. Aloe vera, let it be noted, is nothing short of a botanical miracle worker, revered for the cooling, restorative gel it harbors within its plump leaves, a salve for burns and a soothing balm for skin irritations. Who wouldn't want a natural first-aid kit on their windowsill, ready to provide relief immediately? A gentle leaf tear reveals the healing essence that so many attest to. Another member of this botanical pharmacy is ginger, revered for infusing culinary dishes with zest and heralded for its formidable anti-inflammatory prowess. This gnarly root is reputed for alleviating nausea and joint pain symptoms, highlighting one of the countless gifts offered by Mother Nature's bounty.

Yet, there is always another wonder to unravel. Plant diversity and adaptability continue to be a wellspring of wonder and inspiration. Picture a plant growing unyieldingly in a crevice or perched perilously on a rocky face. Each is a testimony to resilience, a natural tenacity that belongs to this group of life forms, truly deserving of our respect.

Experimenting with Plant-Based DIY Projects

Inspired by these tales of botanical brilliance, why not embark on an adventure that channels this profound reverence into practical endeavors? Engage in plant-based DIY projects and tap into the wisdom these green entities have to offer! Imagine crafting your aloe vera lotion, harnessing its soothing properties to pamper your skin with nature's elegance. Or delve into concocting a spicy, warming ginger tea, a traditional remedy celebrated across cultures for easing an upset stomach and reviving weary souls. These creative experiments will deepen your gratitude for plants and unfurl a spectrum of practical advantages.

Dare to transcend the confines of your abode and immerse yourself in exploring local flora. Visit nearby sanctuaries of green, like parks or botanical gardens, and carefully observe the many plant species that call your region home. Notice their singular characteristics and ingenious adaptations, might you even identify a few phytoremediation mavens among them? Consider maintaining a journal, cataloging your observations and insights, or sketching the intricate and intriguing details of the specimens that draw your gaze.

Such experiential learning encourages a more intimate and insightful connection to the verdant world and enriches one's comprehension of its intricate and expansive capabilities. Herein lies an opportunity to draw directly from nature's vast knowledge repository and grow fluent in applying these teachings in creative, life-enhancing ways.

This vivid tapestry of life envelops us, where each plant holds secrets awaiting discovery. Whether through eager experimen-

CHAPTER 2

tation with new projects or observing their boundless feats, there is more to uncover regarding these green companions with whom we share this Earthly domain. So, adopt the mantle of the plant detective within and embark on a journey to unravel the mysteries within the leaves, stems, and stories of the verdant beings around you!

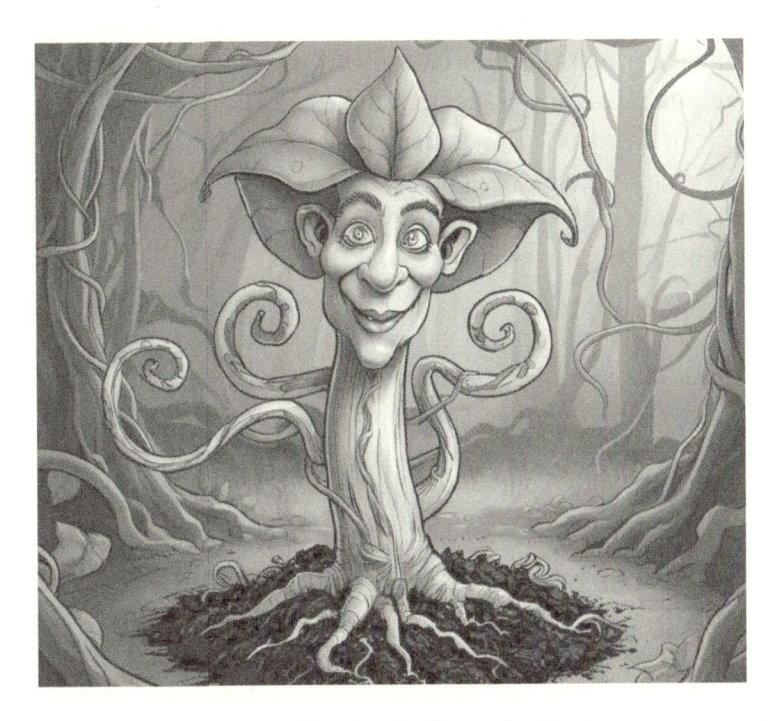

Historical Plant Legends: Stories from the Past

Picture this vivid scene: a plant so entrenched in mystery and enigma that it made the inhabitants of the Middle Ages tremble at its whisper across the wind. Behold the mandrake, a plant with a gnarled root that eerily echoes the human form, filled with limbs and contorted features in its twisted growth. Steeped in ancient lore, the mandrake was said to wield immense magical powers, its essence entwined with the supernatural. Legends claim that the mandrake could unleash a scream so deadly when uprooted that it would strike fear into the hearts of anyone nearby. To thwart its lethal cry, people concocted ingenious methods involving dogs tying a rope to a loyal canine and covering their ears. At the same time, the unsuspecting animal pulled the plant from the earth. Fact or fiction, the mandrake's storied reputation for magic continues to captivate, serving as a timeless reminder of humanity's fascination with and sometimes fear of the arcane and mysterious qualities that plants have held through the ages.

Another splendid gem of the botanical world, draped in the rich fabric of history, is the lotus flower, deeply steeped in ancient Egyptian mythology. The enigmatic Egyptians revered this plant, bestowing upon it a revered status as a powerful symbol of rebirth and creation. Mesmerized by the lotus's ethereal beauty, they believed it emerged from the primordial waters as if it were a divine creation, bringing forth the mighty sun god, Ra. The lotus's serene ability to blossom in the muck and mire of muddy waters only added to its majestic status, emblematic of purity and spiritual elevation. This theme was seamlessly woven into Egyptian artistry and iconography, a testament to the flower's resilience as a powerful metaphor for spiritual awakening. As you immerse yourself in garden soil, knee-deep amid verdant flora, let your mind wander to the serene elegance of the lotus, reflecting on its symbolic metamorphosis from the shadowy depths to the brilliance of light.

Moreover, plants have served as compelling actors on the stage of history, profoundly shaping human events across centuries. Consider the captivating tale of tulip mania that overtook 17th-century Holland, where tulips, with their spectacularly vivid hues and singularly unique patterns, became the supreme object of desire for myriad Dutch citizens. This floral frenzy reached a frenzied pinnacle, with tulip bulbs fetching astronomical prices rumored to exceed the cost of grand houses! Yet, like all bubbles that swell beyond their capacity, this one burst dramatically, leaving a trail of financial ruin. Despite its ephemeral nature, tulip mania carved an indelible mark on economic history, standing today as one of the earliest exemplars of speculative trading and market bubbles that fraught markets with risk.

In another corner of the globe, the life-saving properties of quinine revolutionized the battle against malaria, a disease that wreaked havoc on many tropical regions. Derived meticulously from the bark of the cinchona tree, quinine became an indispensable tool in battling this menacing disease, effectively advancing medical frontiers. Its discovery proved a game-changer, enabling European colonization in malaria-endemic areas by safeguarding explorers and settlers from this relentless affliction. Quinine's role in history underscores the crucial part plants have played in propelling human endeavors and crafting pathways to survival and conquest.

Beyond historical influence, plants have long stood as potent symbols across cultures, etching deep-rooted meanings into the tapestry of human society. The olive branch is an emblem that is most enduring and universally celebrated as a symbol of peace. Originating in ancient Greek mythology, associated with Athena, the goddess of wisdom, the olive branch subsequently became a universal sign of reconciliation and truce. Even today, offering an olive branch signifies goodwill and a heartfelt desire to resolve conflicts peaceably.

And who, indeed, can overlook the timeless allure of the rose? With its longstanding association with love and beauty, the rose transcends the bounds of time and geography. From Shakespearean poetry to modern-day romantic tokens on Valentine's Day, roses have eloquently expressed affection and admiration. Their luxuriously velvety petals and intoxicating scent render them unforgettable symbols of passion and desire testament to how profoundly plants can articulate emotions that words might sometimes struggle to convey.

Engaging with plant history invites you into an open window into human culture and shared experiences. Visiting historical sites that were once tender canvases where notable plant stories unfolded offers a tangible link to these captivating tales of yore. Envision yourself standing in fields that once burst with tulips during Holland's floricultural eruption or leisurely walking through an ancestral olive grove where trees still bear fruit centuries after they were planted.

Literature, too, serves as rich soil for exploring plant symbolism. Dive eagerly into works interlaced with botanical motifs and discover how adeptly authors have employed plants to convey deeper meanings and messages. Whether it's the apple in the story of "Adam and Eve" or the potent poison hemlock marking the grim end of Socrates, these narratives and many more unravel humanity's enduring fascination with the natural world.

Reflect deeply on these historical connectivities as you immerse yourself in gardening, whether tending to your verdant patch or leisurely strolling through parks and botanical sanctuaries. Allow yourself to consider how each plant harbors its own poignant story, a narrative eloquently shaped by human interaction over time. This layered understanding enriches your appreciation for plants and their dynamic roles in shaping the physical landscape and humanity's cultural and intellectual contours.

Let the rich tapestry of history inspire your gardening odyssey by incorporating plants with storied pasts into your collection. Whether cultivating fragrant roses to channel eternal romance or nurturing olive trees as living symbols of peace and perseverance, these plants invite you to meditate on their broader cultural significance, a resonance far beyond mere visual allure.

In doing so, you craft a living mosaic that harmonizes past and present. In this personal garden, each leaf unfurls a story deserving of preservation, ready to captivate and enrich the generations yet to come.

The Secret Life of Seeds: From Dormancy to Awakening

Imagine a seed as a tiny package of potential, lying dormant until the moment is just right. It's like nature's version of a treasure chest, waiting patiently for the key to be turned. Within this unassuming shell lies everything needed to create a new plant, just biding its time. Dormancy is a protective state, ensuring seeds don't sprout prematurely during unsuitable conditions. Germination kicks into gear when the proper signals arrive, often a blend of warmth, moisture, and sometimes light. This is where the magic begins. The seed absorbs water, swelling and breaking through its harsh outer coat. Roots shoot downward, anchoring the seedling, while a shoot emerges skyward, seeking light. It's a delicate dance of nature's choreography, where timing and environmental cues orchestrate a symphony of growth.

Seed coats are like the knights in shining armor of the plant world. They provide not only protection but also aid in dispersal. Have you ever noticed how some seeds have intricate designs or tough exteriors? These coats protect the embryo from harsh conditions like drought or cold. Consider the coconut with its fibrous husk, designed to float across oceans, or the winged seeds of a maple tree that twirl gracefully to the ground like nature's helicopters. These adaptations ensure that seeds reach optimal locations for growth, far from their parent plant's shadow. It's an incredible journey where a seed's design directly impacts its ability to thrive and reproduce.

The variety of seed dispersal methods is astonishing, revealing plants' ingenuity in spreading their progeny far and wide. Among the most familiar are wind-dispersed seeds, like those of dandelions, which have evolved fluffy structures, allowing them to drift on the breeze. You've probably blown on a

CHAPTER 2

dandelion puffball at some point and watched as the seeds floated away, a perfect example of nature's hitchhikers catching a ride on the wind. Then there are burrs, those pesky little hitchhikers that cling to your socks or your dog's fur during a walk in the woods. This clever design ensures seeds get transported to new locations, often far from their original site.

Animal-assisted seed dispersal showcases another level of plant cleverness. Some seeds rely on animals to do the heavy lifting, getting a free ride to new territories. Birds might eat berries and deposit seeds elsewhere through their droppings, while squirrels bury nuts that they may or may not remember to retrieve later. This dynamic partnership benefits both parties: animals get a meal, and plants gain wider distribution. It's a win-win scenario that illustrates nature's interconnectedness and the mutual benefits achieved through evolved relationships.

Imagine a global insurance policy for plant diversity. Welcome to the world of seed banks. These repositories safeguard genetic material from countless plant species, ensuring survival against threats like climate change or habitat destruction. The Svalbard Global Seed Vault in Norway is the most famous example, nestled deep within an Arctic mountain. It's like Fort Knox for seeds, providing secure storage for millions of samples worldwide. This vault is a testament to humanity's foresight in preserving our planet's botanical heritage.

Community seed-saving initiatives are making waves closer to home by encouraging local biodiversity and resilience. These grassroots efforts involve gardeners and farmers preserving heirloom seeds and swapping them within their communities. It's an empowering movement that protects unique plant varieties and fosters collaboration and knowledge sharing among participants. Participating in seed-saving activities, you safeguard our agricultural future and create a living legacy for future generations.

Let's shift gears to something you can try starting seeds at home! It's a rewarding experience that connects you directly with nature's wonders. Begin with a simple setup: recycled containers with drainage holes filled with quality potting soil. Place your chosen seeds at the appropriate depth (a general rule is twice the seed's diameter), then water gently but thoroughly. Position your containers in a sunny spot or under grow lights if natural light is limited.

As you nurture these tiny life forms, consider documenting their progress through journaling. Note changes in appearance, growth rates, and any challenges faced along the way. This practice enhances your understanding of plant development and is a valuable reference for future gardening endeavors. Plus, it's immensely satisfying to flip through pages filled with sketches and notes detailing your plants' journey from seed to sprout.

Starting seeds offer endless opportunities for experimentation and learning. Try different varieties and observe how they respond to varying conditions, perhaps one thrives in partial shade while another flourishes under direct sun. Experiment with companion planting by grouping compatible species for mutual benefit, which naturally enhances growth while minimizing pests.

Embrace this opportunity to invite biodiversity into your garden by selecting heirlooms or native species suited to your region's climate and soil conditions. These resilient plants often boast unique flavors or appearances compared to commercially available counterparts, a delightful reward for adventurous growers willing to try something new! As you embark on this journey of discovery through seed starting, relish each growth stage as it unfolds before your eyes.

The process deepens your appreciation for plants and fosters patience and resilience, qualities that spill over into other aspects of life beyond gardening itself. Witnessing how small actions yield meaningful results instills confidence in one's abilities as a gardener and steward of our planet's natural resources.

So go ahead and grab some seeds today! Nurture them with care and curiosity as they transform into vibrant plants ready to grace your garden with beauty and bounty. The journey from dormancy to awakening awaits. Are you ready?

Edible Oddities: Curious Crops You Can Grow at Home

Imagine stepping into your very own verdant haven, a magical garden that does not need the stamps of a passport to deliver exotic and varied flavors directly to your kitchen. In this enticing domain of nature's bounty, we delve into the intriguing universe of unusual, edible plants ideally suited for cultivation in the comfort of your home.

The Intriguing Realm of Sunchokes

Let us begin with the fascinating sunchokes, also whimsically dubbed Jerusalem artichokes. Ironically, these gnarly tubers share no kinship with artichokes and bear no relation to the historical city of Jerusalem. However, their nutty, earthy flavor introduces a distinct twist that peppers up any dish they accompany. Imagine the sunchoke as a quirky cousin to the conventional potato; they share a subtle sweetness, matting impeccably with a crunchy texture to craft something irresistibly unique. You may roast them to a golden crisp, much like you would with potatoes, or, with a delicate hand, slice them wafer-thin for a refreshing addition atop salads. Sunchokes soon reveal themselves as unexpected gems, bringing surprise and delight to your culinary undertakings.

A Glorious Spin on Spinach: Malabar Glory

Venture further to discover Malabar spinach, an unusual heat-loving green that thrives splendidly where orthodox spinach wilts beneath the sweltering summer sun. With lush, succulent leaves and a gentle tang, it effuses flavor, making it ideal for salads, stir-fries, or sautéed with fragrant, buttery garlic. Malabar spinach isn't merely a delectable inclusion to your menu; its appeal extends to the aesthetic, deep green leaves boasting a glossy sheen while vibrant red stems pulse with color. By nestling this plant within your garden, a dual feast unfolds: a visual spectacle and the provision of a nutritious, heat-resistant green.

Rediscovering Ancient Grains: The Amaranth Experience

CHAPTER 2

Turning our attention to the next marvel, let's indulge in the rediscovery of an ancient grain, amaranth, which anchors its place back into modern gardens, and rightly so. This resilient plant, a relic of antiquity, embodies a nutritional powerhouse, densely packed with protein and essential amino acids. An impressive aspect of amaranth is its gluten-free nature and extraordinary culinary versatility. Imagine boiling it delicately like rice to serve a heartening side dish or ingeniously popping it like popcorn to concoct a wholesome snack. Such endeavor promises to enrich and diversify your dietary spectrum, offering both healthy and delightfully flavorful.

The Extraordinary in the Ordinary: Purslane's Surprising Secret

Have you chanced upon purslane? Often mistaken for an unassuming weed, this plant undisputedly emerges as a hidden nutritional champion. Its leaves and stems brim with omega-3 fatty acids and a wealth of vitamins E, C, and beta carotene, rendering it among the most vitamin-rich leafy greens one can cultivate. With an engagingly tart and salty profile, purslane transforms basic recipes, from launching salads to garnishing soups, it flits gracefully, adding zest and character. Once merely tolerated, embrace this underestimated plant; it promises to blossom into a culinary mainstay within your cooking repertoire.

Cultivating with Confidence: From Ground to Gourmet

Venturing into these unique crops necessitates neither exceptional gardening prowess nor a botanist's touch but merely an open heart willing to traverse unexplored culinary realms. For sunchokes, opt for well-drained soil allied with a sunlit space. Planting in early spring heralds an autumnal bounty of tubers to elevate your gastronomic feats. Malabar spinach revels in warmth; hence, plant it as days grow balmy while pairing it with a trellis or support, allowing a vertical ascent and transforming your garden into a vibrant, space-efficient delight.

Amaranth is remarkably forgiving and thrives in most soils with simple, regular watering. Its vibrant flowers not only provide a nutritious yield but also paint the garden with splashes of color. Meanwhile, purslane grows from seeds lightly settled over the soil with unparalleled ease. With a swift flourish, it spreads, yielding a profusion of leaves ready for harvesting throughout the season.

Culinary Invitations: Hosting Gardens of Flavor

Once these incredible crops come to fruition, culinary creativity knows no bounds. Envisage hosting a delightful tasting soirée with your cultivated produce posing as the soirée headliner. Guests savor unique delights like roasted sunchokes or a fiery Malabar spinach salad, broadening not merely your horizons but those of your companions, welcoming all into the intoxicating foray of unusual culinary crops.

As you soulfully compose recipes, traverse international cuisines where these plants have enchanted palates for aeons. Amaranth, historically steeped in Mexican culinary tradition, encourages you to wend your way through trying amaranth tortillas or nutrient-rich soup incorporations. Purslane's role in Middle Eastern dishes beckons it to mingle with fresh tomatoes and cucumbers, crafting a refreshingly spirited salad.

Cultivation and Curiosity: The Joy of Unsaid Knowledge

The joy cultivated through these crops stretches beyond mere taste, and the adventure nurtures newfound gardening experiences beyond the staple repertoire. You glean a nuanced understanding of each plant's growth, patterns, and idiosyncrasies, savoring the rewarding art of nurturing the extraordinary.

Moreover, these obscure plants magnify the eclectic diversity flourishing within the plant kingdom. They are a cherishing reminder of uncharted flavors lying in wait, luring us into unexplored territories. They beckon us to embrace an unrestricted mind and palate, introducing us to a culinary epiphany of boundless potential.

In conclusion, delving into unusual edible plants unfurls dual adventures in gardening and gastronomy, a marvelous journey unlocking audacious new tastes while incrementally enhancing your gardening prowess. Whether enriching your plate with nutty sunchokes or crunching on vibrant, juicy purslane, these crops pledge a delicious array of rewards that gratify both gardener and gourmet alike.

As we conclude this chapter on fascinating flora and their manifold, spectacular talents, heed the gentle reminder that each plant cradles mysteries yet to be unraveled by observantly curious souls. From edible oddities that excite our plates to legends woven into the tapestry of time, plants transcend mere background scenery; they are integral, living participants in our lifeworld.

Await eagerly the ensuing chapter, which will delve into the pragmatic intricacies of embedding these wonders into your stretch of paradise. It is replete with hands-on tips and guidance curated exclusively for you!

Chapter 3

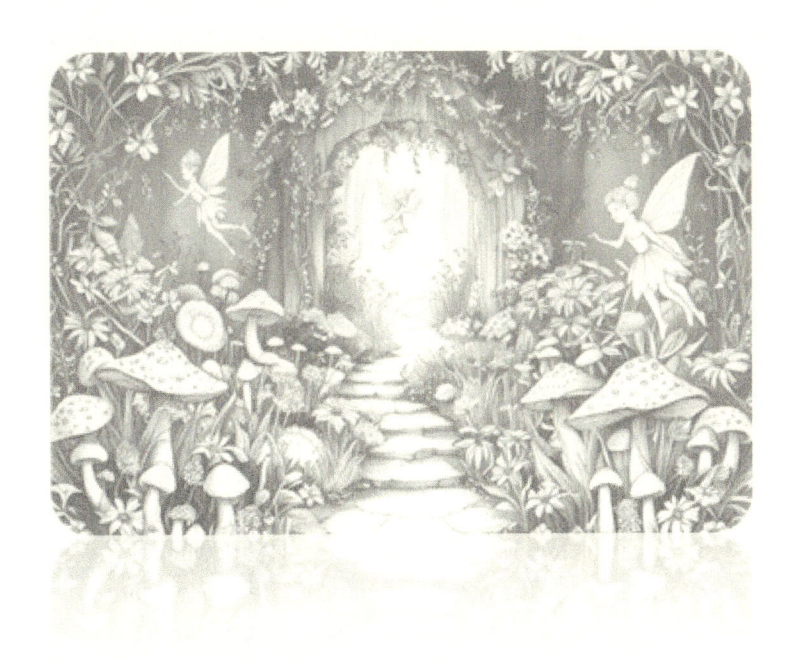

Interactive Gardening Adventures

DIY Fairy Gardens: Enchanting Spaces for Imaginative Play

Imagine, if you will, stumbling upon a miniature world nestled right beneath your feet, where mystical fairies might be flitting wing to petal between colorful blooms, tiny, enchanting pathways guide you to hidden abodes, and a sense of wonder and magic feels just a whimsical stone's throw away. Welcome to the whimsical realm of DIY fairy gardens, a playfully enchanting venture into crafting your own slice of magic right in your backyard or snug little balcony nook. These delightful landscapes aren't just the exclusive domain of children's fantasies; adults often find themselves equally enchanted and almost transported. It's akin to crafting a living storybook that breathes life, grows, and transforms over time, invariably sparking the imaginations of both the young and the young at heart.

To begin weaving this charming miniature magic, consider the actual canvas for your ethereal creation. Shallow pots, artfully broken clay pots, or creatively repurposed containers like whimsical old bowls or rustic baskets work wonders as the foundational base for your landscapes. The chosen container sets the defining stage, marking the scope and boundaries of your tiny magical realm. Don't worry if it's less than perfect; a chipped edge or a strategic crack-adds an element of authenticity and intrigue, hinting at mysterious tales yet untold. Once you've selected your vessel, it's time to breathe life into your enchanted corner! Choose your miniature plants thoughtfully; imagine small succulents, dainty ferns, or velvety mosses that

CHAPTER 3

imitate lush landscapes on a delicate, miniature scale. These plant companions are reasonably low-maintenance, needing minimal upkeep, yet show maximum visual impact.

Next comes the exciting step: you accessorize with abandon, injecting individuality and life into your garden. Miniature furniture, such as tiny benches, gracefully curved swings, or even a petite gazebo, can transform a few square inches into a charming, playful retreat ripe with possibilities. Pebbled pathways invite the eye to wander and explore, creating an illusion of a journey, perhaps toward a miniature house, a cozy secret nook, or even a tiny bridge arching over a little pond. Use tiny figurines of amiable fairies, whimsical woodland creatures, or storytelling elves to breathe vibrancy into your garden. These characters become the pivotal stars of your garden's unfolding narrative, each with its own enchanting adventurers and whimsical tales waiting to unfold and delight your senses.

Speaking of stories, why not inject your fairy garden with vibrant narratives and roles for each character? Envision an elf who steadfastly guards the entrance to a hidden realm or a joyful gnome happily tending to an enchanted vegetable patch. These stories furnish your garden with life by animating its quaint features and providing endless avenues for entertainment and imaginative play. Develop themed sections within your elaborate miniature landscape, perhaps a sun-dappled woodland glen with tiny woodland critters or a tranquil seaside escape complete with sand, shells, and delicate boats. Each section can tell its unique tale or intertwine with others to weave into a larger narrative tapestry resonating throughout the enchanted

space
.

For those inclined toward an eco-friendly and sustainable touch, use natural and recycled materials where possible, allowing Mother Nature to lend her artistry to your creation. Collect twigs during leisurely nature strolls, transforming them into rustic fences, intricate bridges, or elegant arches. Petite stones metamorphose into magical stepping stones or curvaceous borders. Have you stumbled upon an old toy truck or leftover dollhouse furniture languishing in a forgotten corner? Repurpose these into charming garden features. It's sustainable and adds a personal, cherished touch that speaks volumes of your creativity and care. Moss is also an excellent addition; it overlays a natural, plush carpeting that softens harsh edges and bestows an aged, mystical feel upon your darling creation.

Fairchild gardening is special because it warmly invites spirited family involvement. It becomes a joyous, collaborative endeavor that magically brings everyone together in harmony. Assign distinctive roles to each family member. One might specialize in selecting the flora, while another delves into architecting paths and miniature structures, each adding their sprinkle of creativity to create a fascinating whole. Host friendly, jovial competitions to determine who can conjure the most imaginative scene or weave the best story through their personalized garden section. It transcends the realm of simple gardening; it transforms into playtime with the whole of nature as your magical playground.

CHAPTER 3

Reflection Section: Enchanting Exercises

As you embark on this delightful endeavor, take a moment to reflect on these charming exercises designed to enrich your experience:

1. **Imagination Sketchbook:** Before you venture into building, sketch out your envisioned fairy garden design within the pages of a notebook. Specify where wondrous paths will meander, where characters might reside and interact, and what magical aspects intrigue your senses. This provides a fantastic opportunity for your imagination to roam unhindered by limits.
2. **Storytelling Moments:** Pen a short, engaging story about the whimsical inhabitants of your fairy garden. How did they serendipitously come to reside there? What delightful adventures and enchanting escapades await them? Share these captivating tales with friends or family to amplify their engagement and involvement.
3. **Nature Scavenger Hunt:** Embark on a delightful scavenger hunt for natural materials like twigs, stones, and feathers to artfully incorporate into your garden. This magical activity intimately connects you with nature while providing unique, personal pieces for decoration.
4. **Photo Journal:** Capture enchanting photos of your fairy garden as it sporadically evolves. Curate a visual diary or scrapbook that documents changes and growth within the garden and yourself as a nature-loving gardener and imaginative storyteller.

Remember, within the whimsical realms of fairy gardening,

there's no designated right or erroneous approach to building your miniature worlds; it's entirely about unfettered creativity and joyfully engaging with the process. Allow your imagination to function as both guide and companion as you craft these miniature landscapes brimming with magic and wonderment.

In these enchanted spaces, you'll find more than just verdant plants; you'll unearth stories yearning to be unfurled, memories waiting to be crafted, and adventurous scenarios eager to unfold as the days go by. So gather those inviting containers, assemble your eclectic materials, and let's weave some splendid enchantment into our gardens, tenderly casting spells of wonder, no matter how small or towering, into our own corners of the world!

CHAPTER 3

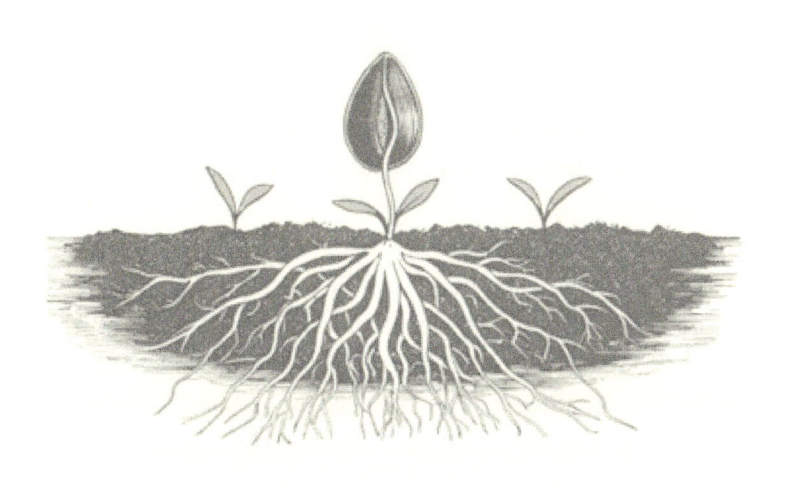

Seed Starting Success: Growing Your First Seedlings

Embarking on the adventure of growing your first seedlings is like opening the door to a world teeming with potential, growth, and budding life. Each tiny seed encapsulates a compact packet brimming with the essence of life, waiting, with quiet expectation, for you to unleash its inherent capabilities. It is the beginning of a journey where you become a caretaker and guide, nurturing nature's wonders into full bloom. Start by thoughtfully selecting well-suited seeds that are suitable for your climate and in harmony with the current season. It's futile planting tomatoes in the chilly embrace of winter unless you dwell in the perpetual warmth of the tropics. Thus, it is wise to check your local planting calendar; it is your guiding map to success in choosing plant varieties that will flourish. Opt for seeds from reputable sources; this ensures quality while providing peace of mind. Moreover, please do not shy away from heirloom varieties; they are often lush with flavor and steeped in history, providing a narrative and nourishment.

Once your seeds are selected, the next step is preparing seed trays and soil mix. A good seed-starting mix is your foundational base that is light, well-draining, and nutrient-rich. You can create your own by combining equal parts of peat moss, vermiculite, and perlite, gently crafting a nurturing bed for the growth to come. Fill your trays with this mix, gently firming it down to dislodge any lurking air pockets. The cleanliness of your tools and workspace is paramount; cleanliness is next to godliness when it comes to seed starting. Proactively sterilize your trays before use. This meticulous act helps prevent damping-off disease, which can transform your seedlings from hopeful sprouts to mushy nightmares.

Illuminating Growth with the Right Light

Lighting is crucial for fostering healthy seedlings. It plays a significant role, akin to the sun bestowing life, in determining the robustness of your plant babies, as they require about 12-16 hours of light daily to grow strong and stocky, staying far from becoming leggy and weak. If you're fortunate to utilize natural light, a south-facing window offers a perfect, sun-drenched wonder that can work wonders. Alternatively, grow lights present a more reliable solution, especially during the darker, overcast months. Position the lights approximately two inches above the seedlings and rub shoulders with flexibility,

CHAPTER 3

adjusting as they grow. Utilize timers to mimic natural daylight cycles, giving your seedlings a dependable, rhythmic routine.

The delicate art of watering requires your utmost attention, competing for complexity with the act of balancing on a tightrope. While it might appear straightforward, it is crucial to know how to keep your seedlings adequately hydrated. Overwatering can be as detrimental as underwatering. Your goal is to find the favorable Goldilocks zone, where conditions are just right. Gently moistening the soil mix before planting your seeds is practiced with patience and precision, followed by sparing watering until germination. A spray bottle proves handy for imparting gentle moisture without disrupting the delicate seeds. After they sprout, watering from the base is ideal, allowing the soil to absorb moisture gradually, climbing upwards, thus averting the potential saturation of tender leaves.

Witnessing the Miracle of Nature Unfold

When those first vivid green shoots courageously burst through the soil, it's like witnessing a miraculous spectacle unfolding in slow motion. It becomes a testament to nature's wonder and your own nurturing skill. However, patience is an invaluable virtue at this stage; prematurely rushing your seedlings outdoors can lead to a shocking demise. Enter the vital process known as "hardening off." This gradual acclimation prepares your seedlings for outdoor conditions. Start by placing them outdoors for a few hours daily, increasing the duration over a week. This valuable exposure toughens them for life beyond the cozy confines of your indoor setup, strengthening their resolve to thrive in the open environment.

Timing is everything in the art of transplanting seedlings. You must astutely wait until the ominous threat of frost has passed and your plants showcase at least two sets of true leaves. Favorable weather, a cloudy day or late afternoon, minimizes transplant shock from direct sunlight. When transplanting, gently tease apart pot-bound roots and position them at the same depth as indoors, except for tomatoes. They relish being planted deeper, encouraging robust root development.

Transplanting is like sending your child off to college; it fosters excitement and dread in equal parts. Once they are comprehensively settled in their new home, a thoughtful offering of water and soothing mulch keeps them cozy. They will extend their roots and aspirations here, growing into robust, flourishing plants.

Cultivate Adventure and Curiosity in Gardening

Encourage an adventurous spirit in your gardening by experimenting with planting diverse seed varieties each season. This diversity breathes intrigue, and every new planting becomes an enticing experiment. Keep a detailed seed-starting journal where you document and reflect on what methods work and what falters, record growth progress, and note any pests or diseases that surface. This living record, teeming with insight, will mature into an invaluable resource over time, guiding future planting decisions and empowering you to learn from moments past.

Don't shy away from variety; infuse your garden with novelty and excitement by trying something new. An unusual heirloom tomato or an offbeat purple carrot will catch your fancy. These

CHAPTER 3

delightful experiments add excitement and may unveil a new favorite, integrating as a perennial staple in your garden for many seasons to come.

A keen sense of observation is indelible in a gardener's toolkit. Through attentive observation, watch for how your seedlings respond to different conditions, tweaking your care according to their thriving needs. Does a bit more sunlight invigorate them, or does a mindful reduction of water suffice? An infusion of extra compost in their soil coaxes more vigorous growth, or a sheltered corner from the wind becomes a safe haven.

By lovingly keeping these observations in your journal, you sharpen your skills as a gardener and simultaneously develop an intimate, profound understanding of each plant's unique needs and personality.

Seed starting isn't merely about growing plants. It symbolizes the nurturing of potential and the witnessing of extraordinary transformations firsthand. It becomes a rewarding exercise in patience and perseverance, ultimately leading to the vibrant greenery and gratifying, delicious harvests that follow.

So, gather those seed packets, shake off the dust cloaking those trays, and prepare yourself for the delightful, transformative journey of growing something spectacular from virtually nothing, one tiny, promising seedling at a time!

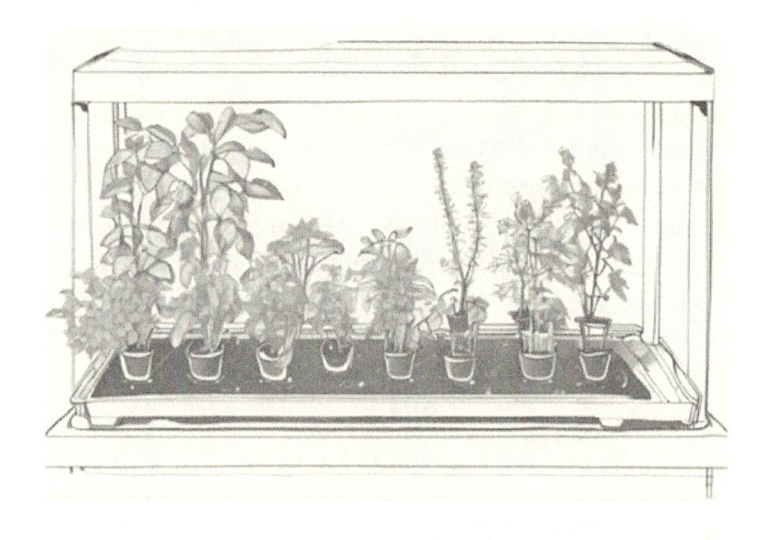

Propagation Playground: Expanding Your Plant Collection

Propagation, in its simplest essence, is the art and science of bringing new life from existing flora, much like whipping up a delicious cake from basic ingredients that you have at home. Instead of reaching for traditional baking essentials like flour, sugar, and eggs, you find yourself collecting bits of plants, cuttings, seeds, or even leaf sections to create vibrant new additions to your garden. This practice allows enthusiastic gardeners to diversify and grow their gardens without the expense of purchasing new plants and provides a deep sense of accomplishment. It's akin to buying a simple stock, only to watch it burgeon into a flourishing investment, doubling or tripling over time. Think of it as nature's buy-one-get-one-free offer. This enriching endeavor invites you to play the role of a backyard scientist, experimenting with various botanical techniques and savoring the satisfaction as life bursts forth from mere snippets of greenery.

Taking Cuttings: Plant Pieces to New Beginnings

Let's start by delving into one of the more straightforward techniques: the artful practice of taking cuttings from herbaceous plants. This method allows you to snip a portion from an established, flourishing plant and coax it to develop its own root system. Begin by selecting a healthy stem that is resilient and not currently flowering. This is crucial as flowering stems often focus more on supporting bloom than developing the necessary roots for propagation. Make a clean cut just beneath a node, those distinctive little bumps or marks on the stem from where leaves or branches sprout. Envision these nodes as the sweet spots on a tennis racket, the perfect point where the energy and potential of the plant are concentrated for your next move.

After making your cut, removing the lower leaves is key. This prevents any unwanted decay when placing the cutting in water or soil. Should you choose to root in water, using a clear glass container is both practical and mesmerizing, offering a peek into the intricate underwater world of root development. Watching roots snake and curl around the confined space is like witnessing a delicate aquatic ballet. Conversely, if soil suits your approach better, ensuring the medium is light and well-draining provides a nurturing environment where new roots can readily establish themselves without being overwhelmed.

Layering: Nature's Way of Doubling Up

Layering is a less intrusive, incredibly resourceful technique for those who cultivate vining plants, such as ivy or the delightful philodendron. Through layering, you can propagate a new plant while it still benefits from its connection to the parent plant until fully autonomous. Continue nurturing the flexible vine as you guide it gently to the ground. By fastening it subtly with a small U-shaped wire or even a modest rock so that it maintains soil contact, you allow nature to take its course. Then, cover the stem with a thin top layer of earth, exposing the vine tip to air. Over time, frequently several weeks, roots will quietly yet efficiently establish themselves along the buried vine segment. Once a robust root system has formed, you can confidently sever it from its parental source, and your new plant is ready to step into the world independently.

Dividing Perennials: A Hands-on Approach to Garden Management

Another pragmatic propagation technique involves the division of perennials, especially when faced with sprawling clumps of hostas or daylilies that seem to spill over one another in your garden beds. Time your divisions for early spring or fall when these plants are not in high growth mode, reducing stress. Using garden tools, gently lift the clump from the earth and remove the surrounding soil to reveal the underlying network of roots. The task of dividing can be done gently by hand or with a sharp knife for tougher cases, ensuring each new segment holds onto enough roots to thrive independently. Replant immediately after division, nurturing each section with ample water to ease their transition into the garden and prevent dehydration.

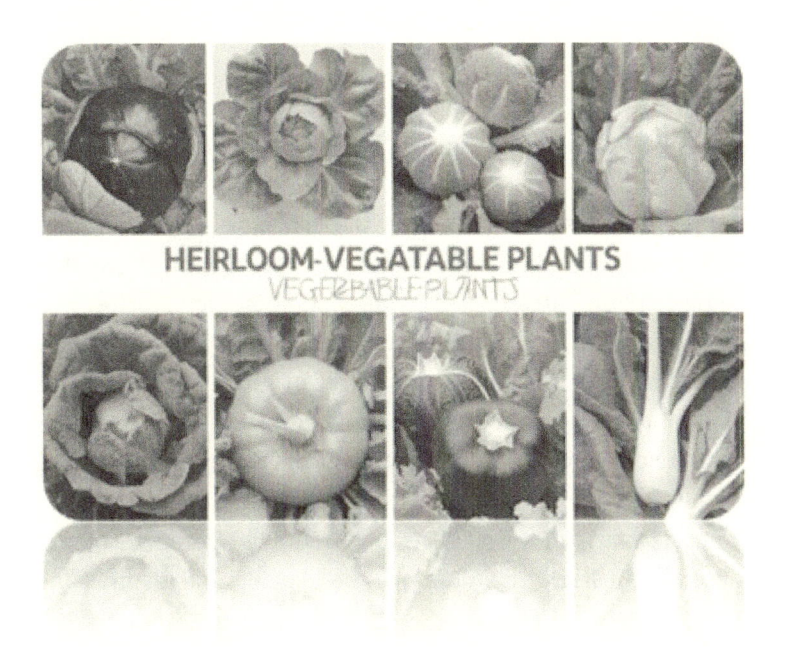

HEIRLOOM-VEGATABLE PLANTS

Preserving Heirlooms: A Propagation Legacy

Propagation extends beyond just expanding your plant collection; it's an opportunity to increase biodiversity and adaptability within your garden's ecosystem in a sustainable manner. Creating fresh growth from established plants saves money and is crucial in preserving heirloom varieties; coveted plant types often missed in commercial outlets. Just like handing down a beloved family recipe, heirloom plants carry their distinctive, historic genetic materials. By championing these heirlooms through propagation, you become the custodian of these cherished greens, fostering their survival and prosperity for future generations.

The Joy of Sharing: Building Connections through Cuttings

Propagation also embodies a spirit of sharing and community. Picture this: a jovial plant swap event where aficionados gather to trade plant cuttings alongside their cherished stories. The atmosphere is exciting with each rare find, like stumbling across an unusual succulent species or gifting a prized fern segment to a neighbor who secretly admires it. It's far more than just an exchange of plants; it crafts community ties and imparts gardening wisdom with each chat and chuckle shared among participants. Such get-togethers swiftly transform into hubs that bustle with vibrant ideas and newfound inspirations.

If in-person interactions prove challenging, online gardening forums and platforms provide excellent venues for connecting with global enthusiasts. Exchange tips on propagation practices, clarify uncertainties and partake in virtual swaps, where cuttings traverse distances by mail, bestowing a touch of your oasis into gardens spread far and wide.

The Delight of Experimentation and Discovery

Propagation begets an atmosphere of curiosity and encourages experimental forays into new practices. It might invite you to try varied techniques to see what unfurls, leading to delightful discoveries that highlight unexpected successes. Such explorations boost patience and a keen eye as you ascertain which strategies align best with particular plant species, cultivating a deeper intimacy with the artistry of nature's unfolding patterns.

As you hone your skills and deepen your understanding, embrace the inevitable trial and error and celebrate the learning that comes from every experiment, whether successful or not. Each instance offers a lesson on different plants' specific nuances and needs. These experiences become your allies, guiding you and your sprawling, lush garden toward a flourishing future.

With propagation in your gardening repertoire, you're not merely multiplying plants; you're nurturing creativity, enhancing knowledge, and building community spirit in equal measure. So venture out with your pruners in hand, seeking out healthy garden specimens, and embark on a propagation journey that promises growth on myriad levels!

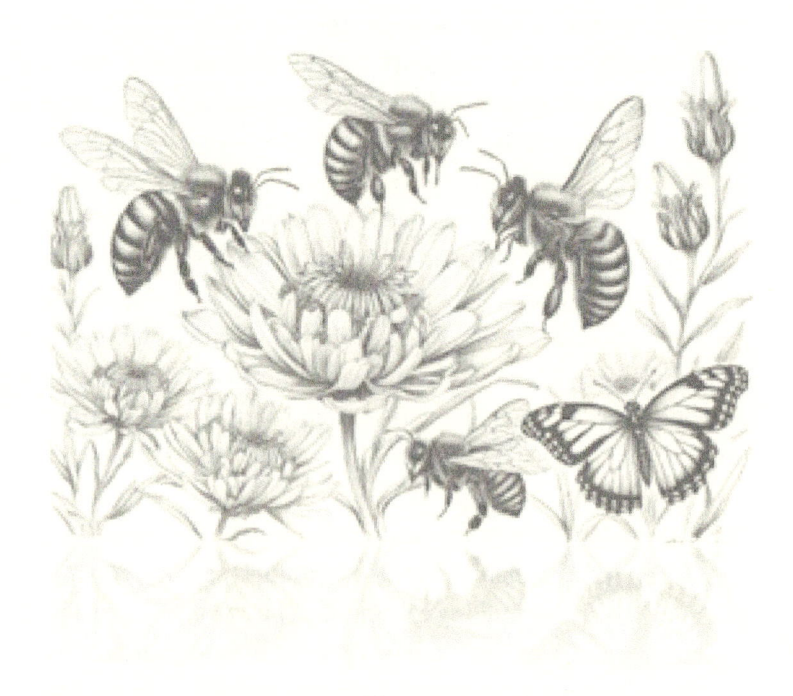

Creating a Pollinator Paradise: Attracting Bees and Butterflies

Imagine your garden abuzz with vibrant life, not simply due to the verdant plants you have carefully nurtured and cherished, but due to the bustling presence of the miniature powerhouses of the natural real pollinators such as bees and butterflies. These small yet mighty wonders play an integral part in the sustainability of our ecosystems, serving as the silent heroes underpinning food production and flourishing plant life. Through their diligent work of pollination, these creatures facilitate the perpetuation of plant species, leading to the generation of fruits, vegetables, and crops essential for survival. Consider

CHAPTER 3

a world devoid of pollinators, where once-bountiful gardens are reduced to sparse patches, stripped of the abundant harvest that feeds our families and surrounds our dining tables.

Yet, the role of pollinators transcends just sustenance; they are pivotal contributors to the richness of biodiversity and the stability of ecological systems. Their presence engenders a dazzling mosaic of life in which myriad species interdependently thrive, buttressing each other and preserving nature's intricate balance. Indeed, their vital activities ensure a harmonious symphony of ecosystems, where each chord and note signifies a different species working together to support the greater harmony of the natural world.

Designing A Pollinator-Friendly Habitat

Designing a garden that welcomes and encourages pollinators is your opportunity to support these tireless agents. Initiating this engaging endeavor begins with cultivating a broad array of nectar-rich blooms that flourish in cycles throughout the year. Through this, you create a consistent cafeteria of nutrients for pollinators, nourishing them across all weather and seasons. Envision it as offering an endless buffet, an enticing display constantly adorned with favorites like coneflowers, zinnias, and lavender. Each of these dazzling and unique blooms calls forth distinct pollinators, so the more extensive your collection of flora, the more varied your garden's visitors will be.

In addition to this remarkable series of floral treats, envisage establishing accessible water sources. A modest, shallow dish, thoughtfully arranged with stones, emerges as a welcoming oasis for bees and butterflies, permitting them a refreshing sip between their tireless fluttering journeys from bloom to bloom. This modest addition can substantially impact these hardworking insects, providing a small respite.

Providing Shelter and Sanctuary

A pollinator haven is incomplete without suitable sanctuaries. Strategic placement of logs or stones can serve as abodes for solitary bees, whereas dense shrubbery offers an impenetrable bastion against predators and adverse weather conditions. Emphasizing native plants within your scheme is vital; these flora need less intervention for upkeep and present familiar refuge spaces that align with local wildlife's natural behaviors and habitats. Infusing these indigenously adapted plants into your green landscape crafts a heartfelt invitation to pollinators, supporting their lifecycle in the region they belong to.

Sustainable Practices for Pollinator Health

As you meticulously blueprint your garden, align your efforts with practices that cherish and prioritize pollinator well-being. Eliminate the use of chemical pesticides that imperil these delicate beings. Opt for organic pest control methodologies such as companion planting or using natural deterrents. This pivotal choice preserves pollinator health and nurtures an overall invigorated garden ecosystem. By selecting native plant species, your gardening becomes less of a chore and more of an alliance with nature, as these plants should ideally flourish with negligible interference due to their natural resistance to pests and ailments.

Participating in Conservation Efforts

Your personal haven can transcend its private serenity to become a facet of a more comprehensive conservation drive. Enrolling in citizen science projects provides meaningful data to researchers examining pollinator demographics and behavior. Keep a detailed log, diligently recording your observations of pollinator visits and activities within your garden. Take note of which blossoms attract the most attention and any patterns or transformations that arise over time. This accumulated information culminates in a treasure trove of insights for scientists intent on unraveling trends, empowering them to compose strategies targeting preservation.

Further, extend your influence by engaging with community conservation undertakings. Various locales have launched initiatives to architect pollinator corridors and interconnected expanses of habitat that permit pollinators to orbit freely and thrive, even amidst urban sprawl. Collaborative efforts with your neighbors or entry into community collectives can bolster the development of these essential pathways, promoting a neighborhood interwoven with pollinator-friendly gardens, each acting as a stepping stone across cityscapes.

Cultivating a Mindset of Stewardship

Imagine a future where neighborhoods brim with sanctuaries for bees and butterflies, urban areas refashioned into havens that reconnect fragmented habitats and bolster diverse species.

Plants alone cannot realize such a vision; it's about nurturing a mindset of stewardship and caretaking for our environment. It is embracing that our gardens enfold a larger ecosystem narrative and that our deeds resonate with effects that cascade far beyond our garden gates.

As we conclude this chapter celebrating interactive gardening odysseys, recollect that each seed tenderly sown, each bee assiduously cultivated, reverberates throughout earth's complex web of life. Engaging in crafting whimsy-filled fairy gardens, fostering tender seedlings, and advancing plant propagation, every mindful decision as a gardener fortifies the vigor and health of our shared planet.

In the subsequent chapter, we will uncover how gardening conveys benefits extending beyond nurturing nature to enriching our lives. We will explore the profound restorative energy of tending to plants and how it holistically increases life gratification. Prepare to embark on this enlightening exploration of cultivating well-being from soil to soul.

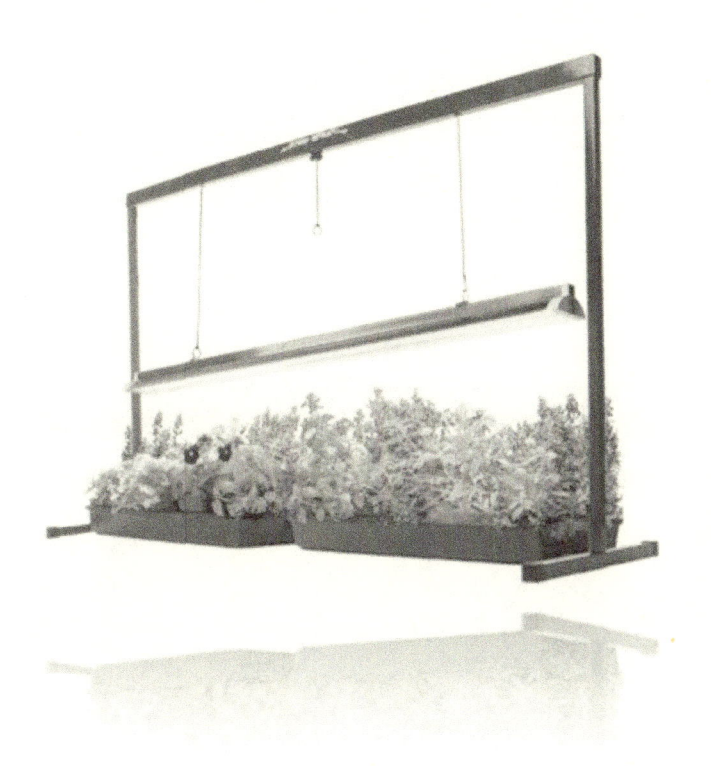

CHAPTER 3

Chapter 4

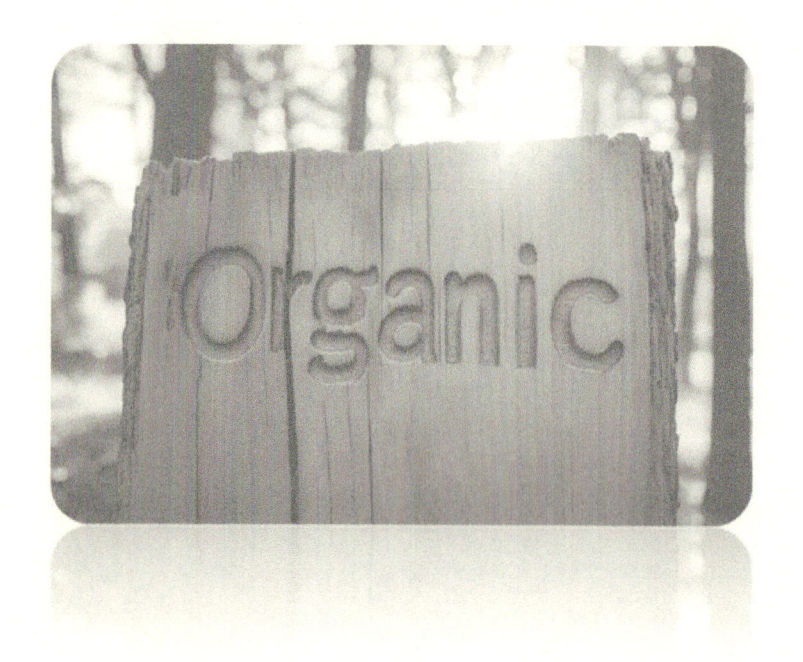

CHAPTER 4

Sustainable Gardening Practices

Organic Gardening: Growing Naturally Without Chemicals

Imagine walking into your garden, greeted by vibrant blooms and lush greens, knowing they've been cultivated without a hint of synthetic chemicals. That's the magic of organic gardening! It's not just a method; it's a philosophy that embraces nature's rhythms. At its core, organic gardening focuses on creating a balanced ecosystem. The emphasis is on soil health and biodiversity, making the earth beneath your feet as alive as the plants. By avoiding synthetic fertilizers and pesticides, you're protecting your plants and nurturing a healthier environment. This approach ensures that your garden thrives naturally without disrupting ecological harmony.

Now, let's talk about pests, those pesky critters that seem to love your plants as much as you do. Instead of reaching for harsh chemicals, consider inviting some beneficial insects to your garden party. Ladybugs, for instance, are like tiny bouncers that patrol your garden, munching on aphids and keeping the peace. Neem oil is another natural ally. Derived from the seeds of the neem tree, it acts as an insect repellent and disrupts the life cycle of pests without harming beneficial insects. Insecticidal soaps, made from plant oils and animal fat, are gentle yet practical solutions to deter unwanted visitors.

Healthy soil is the foundation of any thriving garden. Think of it as the nutritious soup that feeds your plants. To enrich it organically, consider adding compost and well-rotted manure. Compost is like a multivitamin packed with nutrients and beneficial microbes for your garden. It improves soil structure and fertility, ensuring your plants have everything they need to grow strong. Green manures and cover crops also play a starring role in soil health. When grown and then tilled back into the soil, they act as natural fertilizers, adding organic matter and nitrogen to the earth.

Imagine having a wholesome garden that could earn a badge of honor and enter organic certification. While this process might seem daunting, it comes with significant benefits. Understanding organic labeling gives you an edge in the marketplace by making your produce more appealing to eco-conscious consumers. This certification assures buyers that your fruits and veggies are chemical-free and grown sustainably. The market appeal of organic produce is undeniable, often fetching higher prices due to its perceived health and environmental benefits.

Interactive Element: Natural Pest Control Checklist

1. **Introduce Beneficial Insects**: Attract ladybugs and lacewings with flowering plants like dill and fennel.
2. **Use Neem Oil**: Spray neem oil on affected plants early in the morning or late afternoon.
3. **Apply Insecticidal Soaps**: Use these soaps on soft-bodied insects such as aphids for best results.
4. **Encourage Natural Predators**: Install birdhouses to attract insect-eating birds.
5. **Rotate Crops**: Prevent pest buildup by changing planting locations each season.

CHAPTER 4

By implementing these organic practices, you create a sustainable garden that thrives in harmony with nature. Each small action contributes to a more significant impact: healthier plants, richer soil, and a vibrant ecosystem teeming with life. As you embrace organic gardening, you'll find a deeper connection to the land, a sense of stewardship over the environment, and a garden that's not just beautiful but bountiful.

It's about cultivating resilience and diversity, creating a peaceful haven where plants and pollinators coexist. This chapter invites you to explore new possibilities in gardening without chemicals. As you dig deeper into organic practices, you'll discover that nature provides all the tools to maintain balance and nurture growth. So grab your trowel, and let's turn that plot of earth into an organic oasis where everything flourishes naturally!

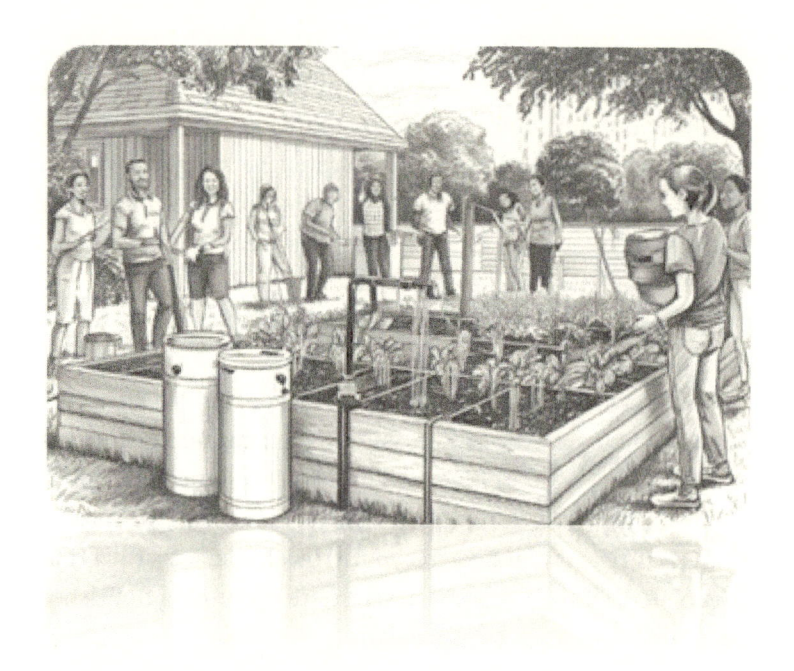

Water-Wise Gardening: Techniques for Conservation

Water is vital for life, and your garden isn't any different. As droughts become more frequent and water scarcity looms, conserving this precious resource becomes crucial. Reducing water usage in your garden helps the environment and keeps your water bills in check. It's a win-win! By conserving water, you maintain local ecosystems, ensuring that rivers and lakes remain full for wildlife and other uses. While the impact of droughts can be devastating, you have the power to mitigate their effects with wise gardening choices.

To start, let's chat about some efficient irrigation methods. Drip irrigation systems are like the VIP treatment for your plants.

CHAPTER 4

These systems deliver water directly to the root zone, minimizing evaporation and runoff. It's precision watering at its finest. Soaker hoses are another fantastic option. They slowly release water along their length, ensuring even moisture distribution in your garden beds. Both techniques maximize water use, keeping your plants happy while conserving resources. Plus, they save you time on your watering routine.

Why let rainwater go to waste when you can harness its power? Rainwater harvesting is an eco-friendly way to quench your garden's thirst. Installing rain barrels is a simple step that makes a big difference. These barrels collect runoff from your roof, storing it for future use during dry spells. You can use this natural bounty to water your garden, reducing reliance on municipal water supplies. Designing rain gardens takes it up a notch by creating natural basins that capture rainwater, allowing it to infiltrate the soil and recharge groundwater slowly.

Choosing the right plants is key to a water-wise garden. Drought-tolerant species thrive with minimal hydration, making them perfect candidates for conserving water. Succulents are the poster children of low-water gardening. With their fleshy leaves and unique forms, they store water like camels in the desert. But don't stop there! Consider xeriscaping plants adapted to arid conditions that bring beauty and resilience to your landscape. Native species are also champions of water conservation. They've evolved to thrive in local climates, requiring less irrigation while supporting local wildlife.

Picture a garden where each drop of water counts, where plants are perfectly adapted to make the most of every sprinkle. This isn't just a fantasy; it's achievable with thoughtful planning and plant selection. Imagine strolling through a lush landscape filled with native grasses swaying gently in the breeze, their deep roots easily tapping into groundwater reserves. These hardy plants stand resilient against drought, their natural beauty shining even in the hottest months.

As you cultivate your garden oasis, consider how your choices ripple beyond your fence line. By opting for sustainable practices and selecting the right plants, you reduce the demand for local water resources while promoting biodiversity. It's about embracing nature's wisdom and letting it guide your gardening endeavors.

Every decision, from installing a rain barrel to choosing drought-tolerant plants, contributes to a more sustainable world. Water-wise gardening isn't just a trend; it's necessary in our changing climate. By prioritizing conservation and sustainability in your garden, you're taking meaningful steps toward preserving our planet for future generations.

Embrace the challenge of creating a water-efficient garden that thrives with minimal input and maximum impact. Who knew saving water could be so rewarding? As you explore these techniques, you'll discover that a little effort goes a long way in making your garden an eco-friendly haven.

So grab those drip lines, set up that rain barrel, and watch as your garden flourishes with less water and more joy. You're not just growing plants; you're growing a movement toward sustainability and mindfulness in gardening practices. With each droplet saved, you're making a difference in one garden at a time!

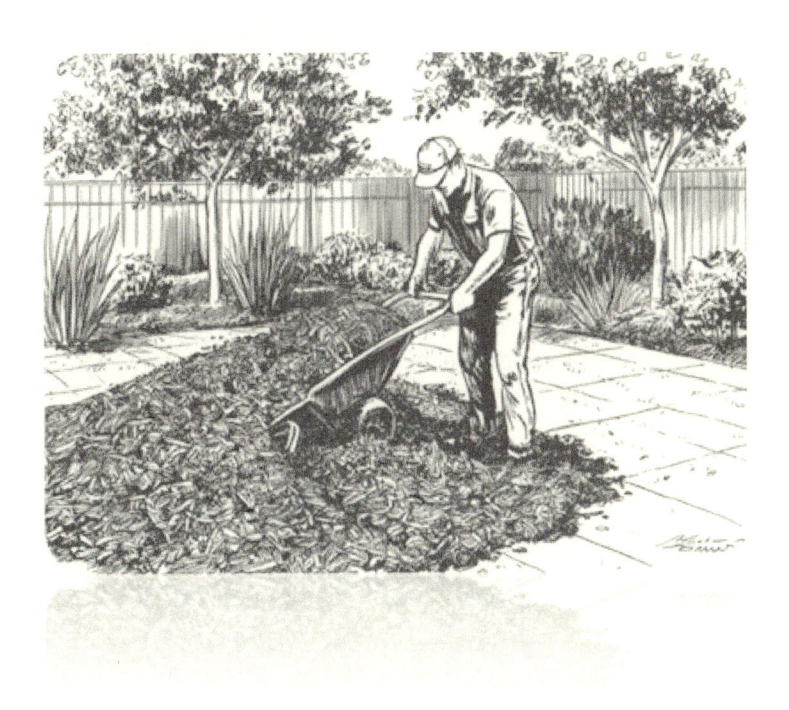

Mulching Magic: Protecting and Enhancing Your Soil

Mulching is like tucking your garden in with a cozy blanket, keeping it snug and happy all year round. It's one of those practices that pulls double duty: it nurtures your plants while saving you time and energy. By spreading a layer of mulch over your soil, you lock in moisture, ensuring your plants have a reliable water supply even during dry spells. This layer is a formidable barrier against weeds, preventing them from sprouting and competing with your cherished blooms for nutrients. Imagine waving goodbye to those pesky intruders without bending backward to yank them out every other day.

Mulch is also a pro at regulating soil temperature. It keeps roots cool during sizzling summer days and shields them from winter's icy grip, like that friend who always knows exactly what to say to keep things mellow. Over time, as organic mulch materials break down, they enrich the soil with nutrients, boosting your garden's productivity and health. A thriving garden isn't just a feast for the eyes; it's a testament to the invisible teamwork happening beneath the surface.

Speaking of mulch materials, you have a smorgasbord of choices. Organic options like wood chips and bark mulch are popular for their natural appeal and effectiveness. They slowly decompose, feeding the soil with organic goodness. Straw and grass clippings are fantastic options, especially if you want something lighter on the wallet. Not to mention, using grass clippings is an excellent way to recycle yard waste. Consider inorganic materials like gravel or black plastic if you prefer something less prone to breaking down. They offer durability but don't provide the same nutrient-boosting benefits as organic mulches.

When applying mulch, a little know-how goes a long way. Aim for a mulch layer about two to four inches thick. Too thin, and it won't suppress weeds; too dense, and you risk suffocating your plants. Avoid piling mulch directly against stems or trunks; it can lead to rot and invite pests. Timing is everything, too. Spring is a prime time to lay down mulch, just after the soil has warmed up but before the weeds have had their chance to invade. Another round in the fall helps protect roots over winter, ensuring your garden bounces back with vigor when spring arrives.

But who says mulch has to be all business and no fun? Why not use it as an artistic element in your garden design? Create patterns with different colored mulches or design pathways that lead visitors on a whimsical journey through your blooms. Decorative mulch can add texture and contrast, highlighting specific features or creating focal points in your landscape. Picture a winding path of crushed shells or a mosaic of pebbles catching the sunlight between flower beds. With some creativity, mulch transforms from a practical necessity into an integral part of your garden's aesthetic allure.

Visual Element: Mulch Design Inspiration Chart

1. **Patterned Pathways**: Use contrasting mulch colors to create patterns or geometric designs.
2. **Textured Borders**: Experiment with different textures—bark chips next to smooth stones.
3. **Color Blocking**: Use dyed mulches to match or contrast flower colors.
4. **Feature Frames**: Highlight focal plants with a distinct mulch border.
5. **Whimsical Spirals**: Lay out spirals or waves for visual interest.

THE GARDEN GUIDE "FUN FACTS FOR BUDDING GREEN THUMB'S"

Mulching is more than just covering dirt; it's about creating an environment where plants can thrive with minimal fuss and maximum effect. Choosing the right materials and techniques can boost productivity while reducing maintenance—a gardener's dream! Plus, you'll add visual flair to your space with creative designs that draw admiration from visitors and enviable glances from neighbors.

So next time you're out in your garden, consider giving it the mulching makeover it deserves. Your plants will thank you by flourishing beautifully, and you'll appreciate the reduced workload and enhanced aesthetics that come with it!

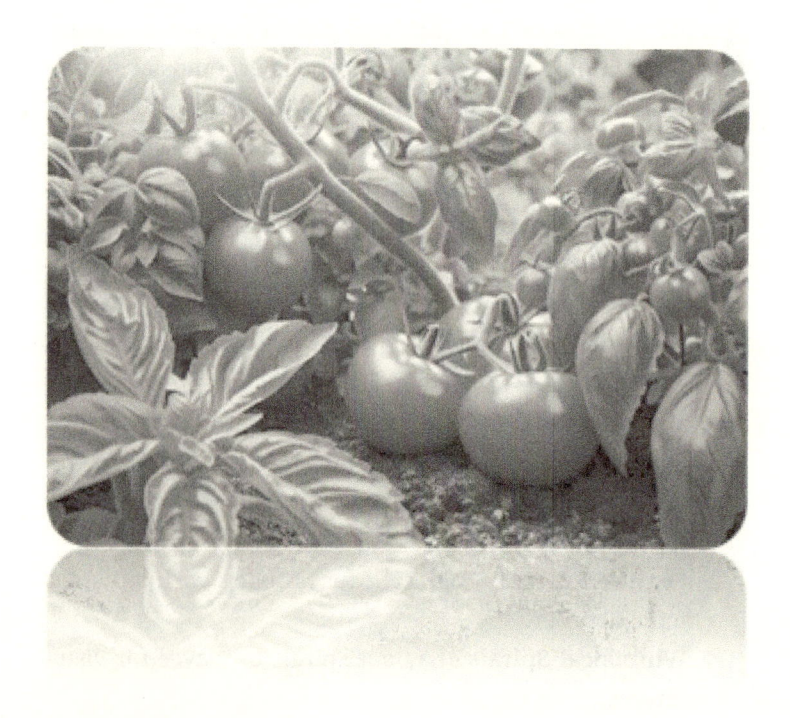

CHAPTER 4

Companion Planting: Boosting Growth and Pest Control

Imagine a garden where plants have perfect buddies—partners that support each other's growth, ward off pests, and invite helpful insects to hang out. That's the charm of companion planting. It's like matchmaking for your garden, where the right pairings lead to a thriving, harmonious environment. Some plants get along better together, enhancing each other's health and growth through beneficial interactions. With companion planting, you can strategically select plant combinations that complement one another, creating a dynamic ecosystem that thrives on natural synergies.

Take tomatoes and basil, for instance. They're the Bonnie and Clyde of the garden world, inseparable and mutually beneficial. Basil enhances the flavor of tomatoes and repels insects like thrips and aphids. Meanwhile, carrots and onions are another stellar duo. Onions release a pungent aroma that deters carrot root flies, while carrots help loosen the soil around onions, allowing them to grow more freely. These partnerships don't just happen by accident; they're based on natural plant chemistry and centuries of gardening wisdom.

The science behind companion planting is fascinating. Some plants release chemicals called allelochemicals that can inhibit the growth of neighboring plants, an effect known as allelopathy. However, these allelochemicals can deter pests or enhance growth when used wisely. Legumes like peas and beans are fantastic companions because they fix nitrogen in the soil, enriching it for their plant buddies. Their roots host nitrogen-fixing bacteria that convert atmospheric nitrogen into a form plants can use, making them excellent partners for heavy feeders like corn or brassicas.

Planning a garden with companion planting in mind requires a little strategy. Start by mapping out your garden layout, considering the space each plant needs to grow and their light requirements. Group compatible plants together and avoid placing antagonistic plants near each other. For instance, keep fennel away from most vegetables as it inhibits their growth. Rotating crops annually is crucial for maintaining soil health and preventing disease buildup. It disrupts pest life cycles and minimizes nutrient depletion, ensuring soil remains fertile and productive.

To successfully design a companion planting layout, consider the height and spread of your plants. Tall plants like sunflowers can provide shade for heat-sensitive companions like lettuce. Meanwhile, vining plants such as cucumbers can be trained to climb vertical supports, maximizing space and reducing competition on the ground. Interplanting flowers like marigolds or nasturtiums adds beauty, attracting pollinators and beneficial insects. These colorful blooms also serve as sacrificial plants, luring pests away from your main crops.

Incorporating companion planting into your gardening routine is like hosting a well-planned dinner party where every guest complements one another. It encourages diversity and resilience, creating a balanced ecosystem that thrives naturally without synthetic interventions. As you experiment with different plant pairings, you'll discover what works best for your garden's unique conditions. Along the way, you'll learn more about the intricate relationships between plants and how they can support each other in remarkable ways.

By embracing these natural partnerships, you'll transform your plot into a thriving oasis where plants work together harmoniously. Companion planting not only boosts growth and productivity but also fosters a healthier, more sustainable garden environment. As you plan your garden layout this season, consider how companion planting can enhance your gardening experience. With some creativity and observation, you'll unlock the full potential of your garden, one friendly plant pairing at a time.

Embrace the artistry of companion planting as you explore new combinations and witness firsthand how nature's wisdom guides plant interactions. Through thoughtful planning and experimentation, you'll cultivate a garden that's not only bountiful but also resilient against pests and diseases. So grab those seed packets, and let's create a garden where every plant has a friend. Yours will be the envy of the neighborhood!

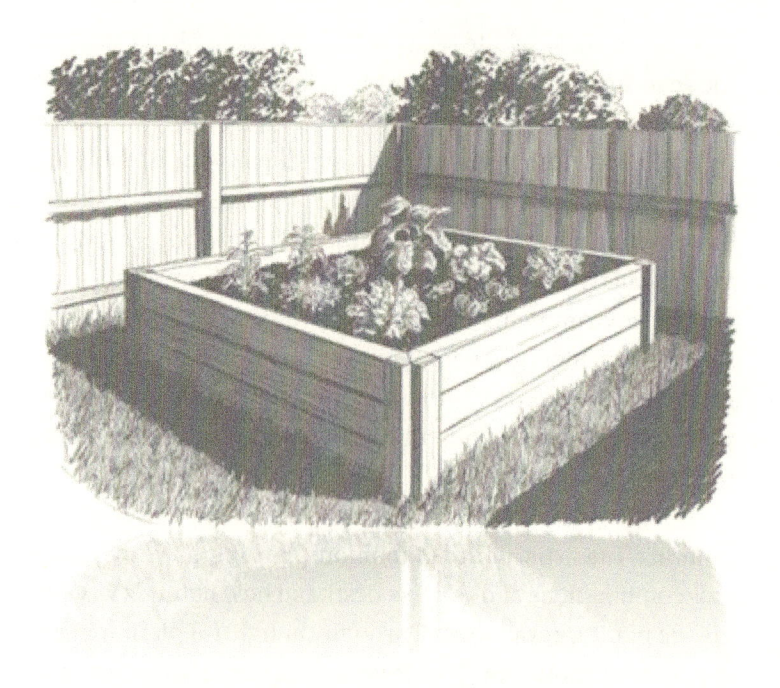

THE GARDEN GUIDE "FUN FACTS FOR BUDDING GREEN THUMB'S"

Building a Raised Bed: A Step-by-Step Guide

Have you ever thought about giving your garden a boost? You're not alone, and raised beds might be the answer you've been looking for. Picture this: they're like the VIP section of your garden, offering features such as improved drainage and enhanced soil quality that are simply unmatched. By strategically raising the soil level, you safeguard against excessive moisture and ensure optimal water flow, meaning roots won't languish in puddles after the heavens open with a heavy downpour. Imagine the relief and vibrancy your plants will show! This thoughtful configuration naturally keeps your plants warmer, helping extend your growing season just that smidgen by a

CHAPTER 4

few weeks, potentially gifting you a more extended period of delightful blooms and bountiful harvests. Plus, don't overlook the ergonomic advantage; raised beds are undeniably easier on the back. You'll no longer need to bend over until you're creaking like an old barn door, thus making gardening an inclusive and joyful activity for everyone, regardless of age or physical limitations.

Feeling eager to get your hands encased in rich, fertile dirt? Fantastic! Let's dive right into the materials necessary for your project. Untreated wood, beloved for its natural aesthetics and availability, is often popular. However, if you're looking to introduce an element of elegance, stone or brick might be your architectural allies. Whichever material you choose, ensure its safety for plants with no noxious substances leaching into your precious soil! Now, take your tape measure and mark out your gardening territory. Opt for a square or rectangular layout; it's easier to manage and maximizes your space efficiently. Moving onto the assembly, you'll want the sides secured firmly. Use screws or brackets to ensure rock-steady stability. If your heart is set on wood, consider lining the inside with landscaping fabric to prolong the structure's life, effectively reducing soil contact and potential decay.

Once you're brimming with satisfaction over your handy construction, it's time for the fun part of filling it up! Start with a foundational layer of coarse material, such as small rocks or gravel. This will help ensure superior drainage. Next, pour in a luxurious blend of high-quality topsoil and compost. This rich concoction provides essential nutrients and substantially improves soil structure. You're crafting a gourmet meal for your plants, laying out a buffet of nutrients right at their roots. While you're at it, incorporate organic matter like aged manure or peat moss. These elements work wonders in maintaining soil health, boosting microbial activity, and providing a nutritional kick.

Now comes the genuinely creative bit! Your raised bed stands before you, like a blank canvas waiting for your artistic touch. Consider introducing trellises for vertical growth—rampant climbers like beans and peas will adore them. Not only do they efficiently save space, but they also introduce a captivating visual element to your garden. Perhaps even build a mini greenhouse cover to shield delicate seedlings from unexpected frost or ever-persistent pests. The colors and materials you choose should ideally complement your existing outdoor space, resulting in a cohesive look that's visually pleasing.

Personalization doesn't stop there. Design aesthetically pleasing layouts by playing with various plant heights, colors, and textures. Strategically place taller plants like tomatoes or sunflowers at the back, allowing shorter ones like lettuce or basil to bask in the unobstructed sun. Add fragrant herbs along the edges for easy access when cooking. It is delightful to reach out and pluck fresh rosemary while concocting a delicious dinner! You can even experiment with arranging plants in creative geometric shapes or spirals for an added element of flair.

Raised beds are more than just functional extensions of the home; they are a tangible expression of your gardening style and creativity. They offer endless possibilities for customization while delivering practical benefits such as improved drainage and enhanced soil quality. Whether your motivation stems from aesthetics or efficiency, keeping these tip top of mind ensures you're well on your way to crafting a thriving garden space that's both breathtakingly beautiful and abundantly bountiful. So dig in and cultivate your artistry, happy planting!

Heirloom Harvests: Preserving Plant Heritage

Heirloom plants are like the treasured recipes passed down from your grandmother, brimming with nostalgia, flavor, and a touch of the past. These open-pollinated varieties have been nurtured and shared through generations, each seed carrying stories of old gardens, family traditions, and cultural history. Unlike their hybrid cousins, heirlooms are not tampered with in laboratories. Their genes remain pure, preserving a spectrum of genetic diversity that modern agriculture often overlooks. This diversity isn't just about aesthetics or taste; it's a lifeline for our food system, offering resilience in the face of climate change and disease pressures.

Growing heirloom varieties in your garden is like planting a piece of history. Start by selecting varieties that suit your local climate and soil conditions. Whether it's a Cherokee Purple tomato with its rich, sweet flavor or a Dragon's Tongue bean with its striking purple stripes, these plants bring character to your garden. Once you've chosen your heirlooms, learning seed-saving techniques is vital. This involves allowing some plants to go to seed, collecting those seeds at the right time, and storing them properly for future planting. It's a rewarding process that connects you to the cycles of nature and the gardeners who came before you.

The benefits of growing heirlooms extend beyond their unique looks. Many gardeners swear by their superior taste and nutritional value. Imagine biting into a juicy tomato that bursts with flavor or enjoying a crisp lettuce leaf that tastes just right. These flavors result from years of careful selection and cultivation by gardeners who prized taste above all. Moreover, heirlooms often boast a natural resilience to local pests and diseases. This inherent toughness means less reliance on chemical interventions, making gardening more sustainable and eco-friendly.

Now, let's talk community. Participating in seed-saving networks is like joining a secret club where everyone's passionate about preserving plant diversity. Local seed exchanges or banks offer opportunities to swap seeds and stories with fellow gardeners. It's a chance to learn from others, share your experiences, and contribute to a legacy of biodiversity. By being part of these communities, you're not just growing plants; you're safeguarding our planet's genetic heritage.

Involvement in these networks also provides access to rare and hard-to-find varieties unavailable in commercial nurseries. It's an exciting treasure hunt where each seed packet promises something special. As you cultivate these heirlooms, consider documenting your journey by photographing the plants, noting their growth patterns, and sharing your results with others. This record serves as a personal keepsake and a resource for future generations.

Gardening with heirlooms is about more than just growing food; it's about nurturing connections. Connections to the past, other gardeners, and the earth itself. Each seed you plant is a step towards preserving cultural history and promoting biodiversity. It's an act of stewardship that benefits not only your garden but the broader ecosystem as well. By embracing heirloom varieties, you become part of a global effort to ensure these unique plants continue to thrive for generations to come.

As we wrap up Chapter 4, remember that sustainable gardening isn't just about techniques. It's about values. It's about cherishing diversity, respecting nature's wisdom, and cultivating a garden that's as kind to the earth as beautiful. In the next chapter, we'll explore how gardening can nourish not just our bodies but also our minds and spirits, turning our gardens into sanctuaries of well-being. Stay tuned as we delve into the holistic benefits of connecting with nature through gardening.

Chapter 5

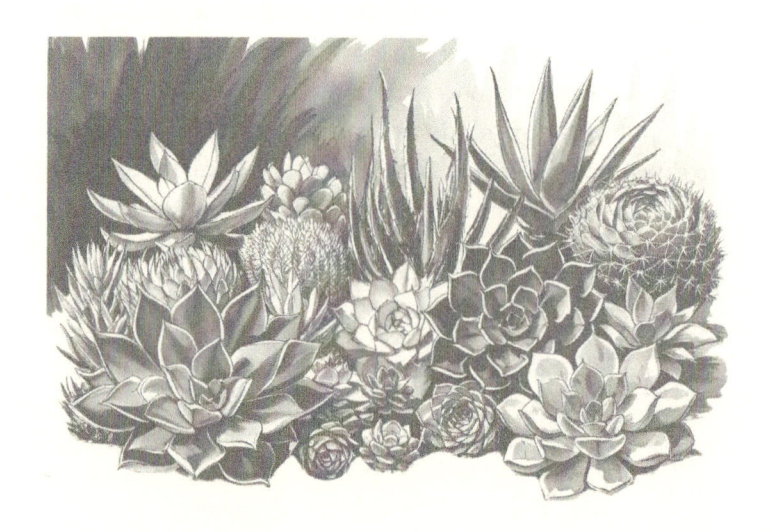

Garden as Art

Creative and Artistic Gardening Succulent Artistry: Designing Stunning Arrangements

CHAPTER 5

Have you ever found yourself entranced, even spellbound, by the breathtaking palettes nature effortlessly paints across the sky at dusk? The play of pinks melting into oranges, which then bleed into deep purples, can leave one longing to capture such an ephemeral moment. Now, allow yourself to dream of encapsulating that essence, not with traditional brushes or pigments, but through the more organic medium of living, breathing plants. Welcome to the enchanting and enthralling realm of succulent artistry, where each plant is both a muse and a masterpiece. Succulents, those resilient wonders of the natural world, showcase a kaleidoscope of shapes, sizes, and hues that rival any artist's palette. Think of them as the unassuming yet radiant stars of the garden, a perfect example of minimal effort yielding maximal beauty. From the intricate mandala-like arrangement of the Echeveria, with its rosette formation unfurling in perfect symmetry, to the seemingly endless cascades of the Sedum, draping gracefully like strands of living gems, succulents offer an inexhaustible reservoir of potential for those who possess the audacity and creative instinct to explore their botanical dreams.

Creating a balanced and visually arresting arrangement with succulents is akin to orchestrating a grand symphony where each note and rest contribute to the sublime harmony of the whole. Consider the firm yet agile structure of a spiky Aloe Vera, which commands attention like the brass section in an orchestra, its tall figure providing a striking backdrop that enhances the softer, more melodious elements around it, such as the gentle, curvaceous leaves of the Echeveria, contributing to the garden's poetic resonance. Contrast breathes life into the arrangement—juxtaposing the smooth fleshiness of certain succulents with the wiry, captivating shape of others or pairing the opulent lushness of some plants with the understated elegance of others. Adding focal points such as a vibrant orange Kalanchoe can serve as the dramatic crescendo within this living composition, capturing the eye and anchoring the visual narrative amid a lush, verdant backdrop. While symmetry often forms the backbone of aesthetics, introducing asymmetry into your design offers a refreshing dynamism reflecting the spontaneity and unpredictability of untouched landscapes.

Venturing beyond the conventional means stepping into a world where your containers invite whispers of wonderment and reminiscence. Reject the mundane in favor of the imaginative and the bold. Picture a hollowed-out log, weathered and rustic, transforming into a cradle for succulents, a vignette of nature meeting nurture. Or dare to repurpose an element from history with a vintage flair, a collection of delicate succulents finding a new home in a series of mismatched teacups or old-world dishware, each piece narrating its own secret, silent stories. These unconventional containers serve not merely as vessels but as integral components of an artistic whole, vehicles for creativity that transform simple arrangements into conversation pieces, each one imbued with personal and artistic significance.

Remember that even the most visually captivating arrangements require regular attention to preserve their splendor. While succulents are famously known for their low-maintenance lifestyle, they possess specific preferences that inform their care. These sun-lovers covet light, thriving best in environments where they can bathe luxuriously in

CHAPTER 5

sunlight for a minimum of six hours daily. However, one must tread cautiously to prevent the cardinal sin of overwatering succulents, which are native to arid regions and have adapted to thrive on sparing moisture. Water sparingly, granting them a thorough soaking every couple of weeks while ensuring the soil dries entirely between indulgences. The well-being of these verdant wonders also hinges on their soil composition; a gritty, coarse blend, to provide excellent drainage is crucial, echoing the conditions of their natural habitats.

Interactive Element: Succulent Arrangement Challenge

With your heart afire and your creative spirit roused, why not take up the succulent arrangement challenge for yourself? Begin by gathering a medley of succulent varieties and a selection of uniquely memorable containers that speak to your artistic inclinations. Experiment and play with different combinations, gently nudging and coaxing them until one arrangement resonates with the depth and harmony you envision. Document your creative journey with before-and-after photographs, personal mementos that chronicle the evolution of your horticultural expression. This exercise is an opportunity to engage in horticultural creativity and an enriching adventure that will leave a lasting imprint on the tapestry of your personal garden narrative.

Succulents offer more than just green foliage; they are a vibrant invitation to delve into the uncharted territories of your imagination. Whether they adorn a sun-drenched windowsill with their warm presence or serve as conversation-sparking centerpieces at a garden gathering, these adaptable gems will inevitably captivate and capture admiration. As they mature and evolve, they manifest as living icons of your creative odyssey, a testament to the beauty that can blossom when human ingenuity meets raw nature. So, as the clay of the earth invites your handiwork, embrace the challenge of succulent artistry; who can foretell what wondrous landscapes your expanded, imaginative vision might uncover?

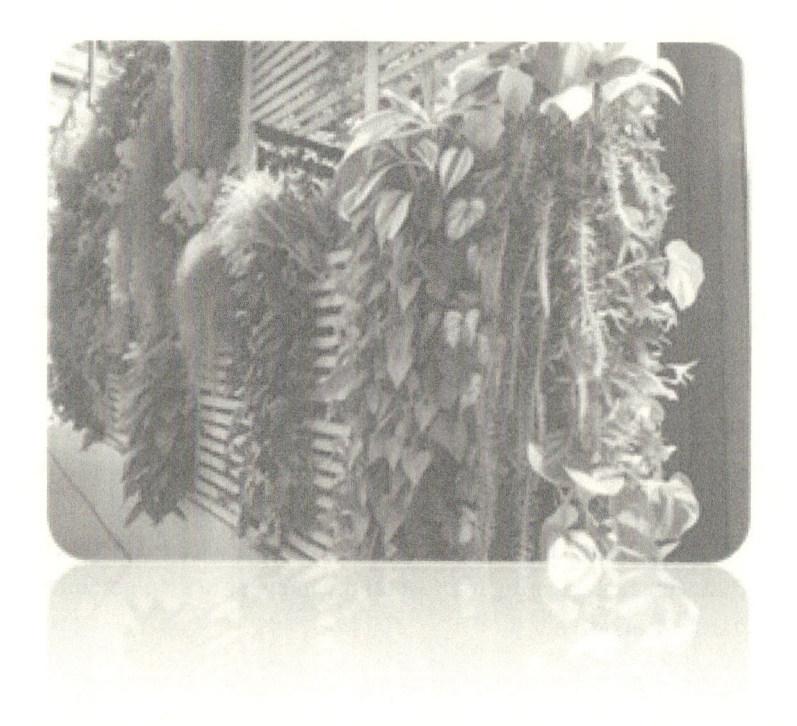

CHAPTER 5

Vertical Gardens: Elevating Your Green Space

Picture this: a cascade of green leaves flowing down a wall or a burst of colorful blooms reaching toward the sky, creating a vertical masterpiece that transforms even the smallest patch of earth into a lush paradise. Vertical gardening is your secret weapon for turning limited space into a thriving oasis. It's like giving your garden a pair of stilts to reach new heights. This technique is a game-changer for anyone working with cramped quarters or those wanting to add privacy with living walls that double as stunning visual displays. Imagine a privacy screen made of vibrant foliage that shields your patio from prying eyes and becomes the talk of your next garden party. By utilizing vertical space, you maximize your garden's potential, making every square inch work overtime in the most beautiful way possible.

Creating a vertical garden structure might sound daunting, but trust me, it's simpler than you think. Start with something as basic yet effective as a pallet garden. These wooden frames can be propped against a wall or stood upright to host an array of herbs, flowers, or even vegetables. Add some landscaping fabric to the back and sides to hold the soil in place, and you're ready to plant. If you feel more ambitious, wall-mounted planters offer a sleek, modern approach. Choose sturdy containers to securely attach to walls or fences, then fill them with your favorite trailing plants. Trellises are another fantastic option, supporting climbing plants that love to stretch their limbs toward the sun. The beauty of these structures is their versatility; they can be customized to fit any space, big or small, and give your garden an architectural flair.

When selecting plants for your vertical garden, think about what thrives in such environments, such as plants that enjoy hanging out. Ferns are an excellent choice; they add lush greenery and tolerate varying light conditions. Trailing vines like pothos bring an elegant drape to your setup, their tendrils weaving through the air like nature's own tapestry. For those who want a taste of freshness right off the wall, strawberries are perfect pocket pals. Imagine plucking a juicy berry while enjoying a morning coffee outside. Dwarf tomatoes also make delightful additions, their compact size lending well to confined spaces while offering bountiful harvests.

Now, let's talk about keeping these vertical wonders happy and healthy. Watering can be tricky with vertical gardens since gravity pulls moisture downward, leaving top plants thirsty and bottom ones drenched. Consider installing a drip irrigation system or strategically placing water reservoirs at different heights to ensure even distribution. You'll want to monitor light exposure diligently; some plants might hog all the sun, leaving others in the shadows. Rotate planters so everyone gets their fair share of sunlight and air circulation. Remember that vertical gardens are living walls, literally—and need breathing room like any other organism.

One of the most rewarding aspects of vertical gardening is watching your creation evolve over time. It's never static; it's a living canvas that changes with the seasons and grows alongside you. As plants mature and fill out their spaces, you'll notice color, texture, and form shifts that keep the garden dynamic and exciting. This constant transformation offers endless opportunities for learning and experimentation. You

CHAPTER 5

may find that certain plant combinations work better than others or discover new techniques for optimizing growth in vertical settings.

Vertical gardens also have a delightful element of surprise. Because they occupy multiple levels, they invite exploration and curiosity. Visitors will find themselves drawn closer, peering at each layer to uncover hidden blooms or unexpected details tucked between leaves. It's like having a secret garden within your main garden, a place where discovery happens around every corner.

And let's not forget about the benefits beyond aesthetics! Vertical gardens can significantly improve air quality by acting as natural air filters, a bonus for urban dwellers dealing with pollution or stale indoor environments. They can also help insulate buildings from temperature fluctuations, reducing energy costs by keeping interiors cooler in summer and warmer in winter.

So there you have it: vertical gardening is more than just stacking plants on top of each other; it's an innovative approach to gardening that combines functionality with artistry. Whether you're looking to make the most of limited space or simply seeking ways to enhance your outdoor living area creatively, elevating your green space through vertical gardens offers endless possibilities brimming with potential and promise.

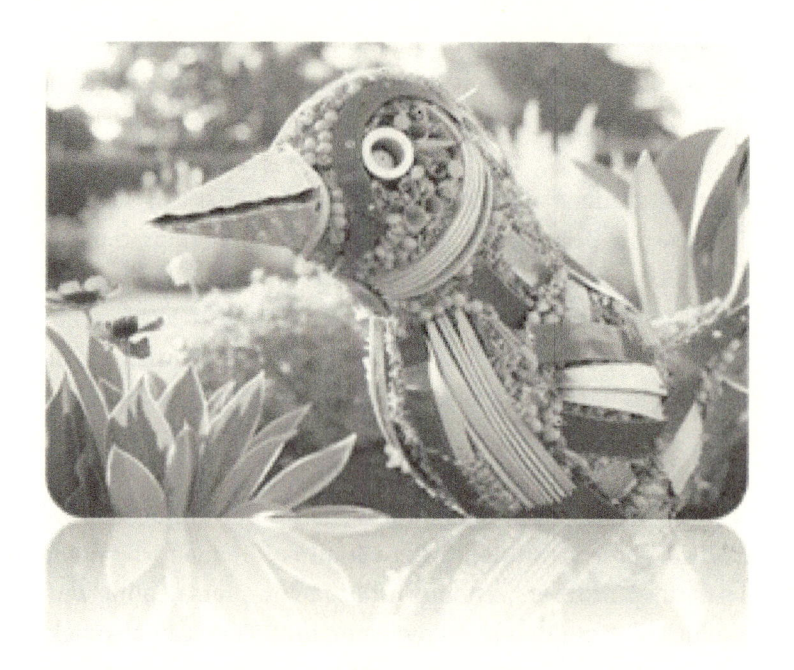

DIY Garden Sculptures: Adding Personal Flair

Imagine your garden as a blank canvas, waiting for your unique touch. Think of it as an outdoor art gallery where every piece reflects a story. Sculptures crafted by your hands can breathe life into this space. Consider using natural elements like stones and wood to create art that blends seamlessly with the landscape. A stack of smooth river stones can transform into a cairn, a simple yet striking tower that guides the eye through your garden. These stone structures can become symbols of balance and patience, offering a sense of tranquility and direction. Meanwhile, wood has a rustic charm all its own. Imagine driftwood, weathered and worn, shaped into organic forms that echo nature's artistry.

CHAPTER 5

For those with a penchant for the unconventional, metal and repurposed objects open up a world of possibilities. Old bicycle wheels can morph into whimsical sculptures, catching the sunlight as they spin gently in the breeze. Rusted gears or pipes, once discarded, find new purpose as abstract creations that add an industrial edge to your garden. Incorporating these elements not only sparks creativity but also gives new life to forgotten materials. It's a form of artistic recycling that celebrates both innovation and sustainability.

Now, let's get hands-on with some beginner-friendly projects. Creating stone cairns is a fantastic start, simple yet satisfying. Gather stones of varying sizes, balancing them carefully to form towers that stand proud against the horizon. Each stone is like a word in a sentence, contributing to the overall story you wish to tell. If you're feeling adventurous, try your hand at fabricating wire sculptures. Bend and twist wire into graceful shapes or playful mobiles that dance in the wind. These can hang from tree branches or stand alone as focal points within your garden.

Themes and motifs serve as the backbone of any great art piece, including garden sculptures. Consider wildlife-inspired designs that bring your garden to life with birds poised for flight or butterflies frozen mid-flutter. These sculptures can transform your garden into a sanctuary for nature lovers. Alternatively, abstract forms offer a modern twist, encouraging viewers to interpret the meaning behind each piece. Bold lines and geometric shapes create an avant-garde atmosphere that can elevate any green space.

Strategic placement is key to integrating sculptures seamlessly into your garden design. Consider framing views with art and place a sculpture at the end of a path to draw visitors deeper into the garden. This acts like punctuation at the end of a sentence, providing closure while inviting exploration. Alternatively, use sculptures to create focal points amid plant arrangements, drawing attention to specific areas or features. Balance is crucial; ensure that your art enhances rather than overwhelms the natural beauty of your plants.

The interplay between art and nature is where magic happens. You inject personality into your garden by adding personal flair through DIY sculptures. Each piece becomes an extension of yourself, a reflection of your creativity and vision. As you wander through your garden, these sculptures become companions on your journey, whispering stories and sparking inspiration.

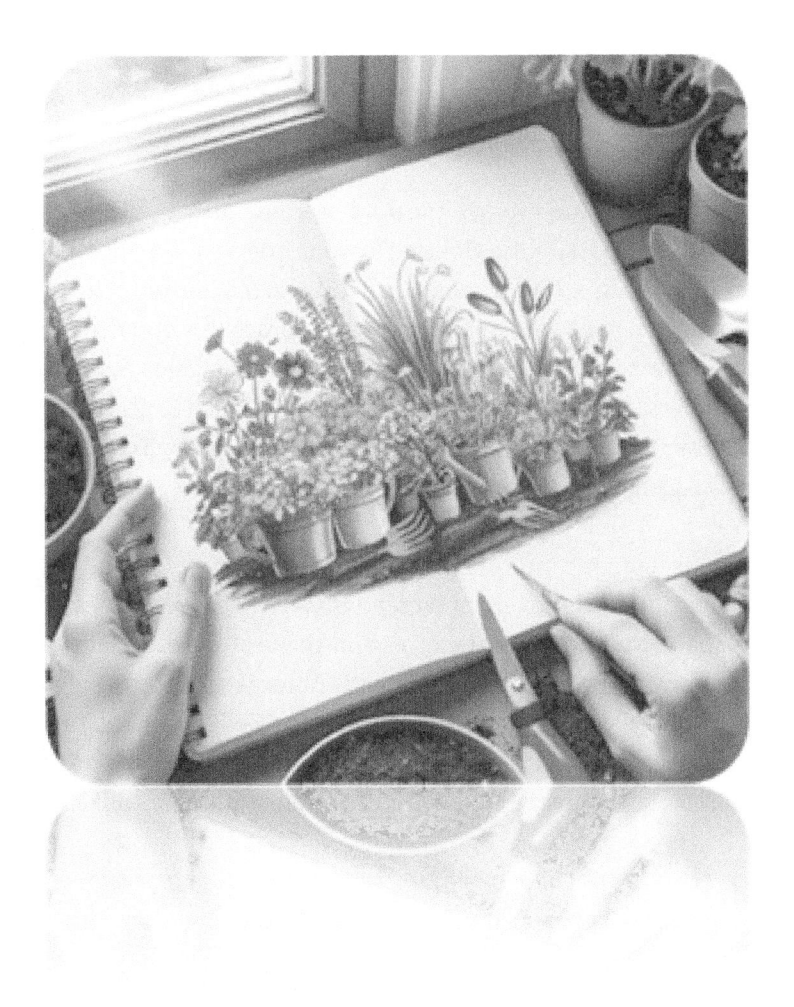

Reflection Section: Artful Garden Journal

Start an artful garden journal to document your creative process. Sketch ideas for sculptures before bringing them to life, capturing the evolution from concept to creation. Use photographs to record progress, noting changes in light and shadow throughout the day. Reflect on how each piece interacts with its surroundings and contributes to your garden's overall harmony.

As you delve into this artistic pursuit, remember there are no rules, only possibilities limited by your imagination. Whether crafted from stone, wood, or metal, each sculpture adds a chapter to your garden's narrative. Embrace this opportunity to express yourself through art that grows alongside nature's wonders. Your garden becomes more than just a collection of plants; it transforms into an ever-evolving masterpiece where beauty knows no bounds.

In this dynamic interplay between art and nature lies endless potential for discovery and creativity. Your garden becomes a space where personal expression thrives—a testament to human ingenuity intertwined with natural splendor. So go ahead, let your imagination run wild! Delight in creating sculptures that enrich both soil and soul, where every curve tells its tale under sun-kissed skies or moonlit nights alike.

Edible Landscaping: Combining Beauty and Function

Imagine walking through a garden where every plant not only pleases the eye but also delights the palate. This isn't a fantasy; it's the world of edible landscaping. It's about blending the aesthetics of ornamental plants with the practicality of food-producing flora, creating a beautiful and bountiful garden. Picture fruit-bearing trees like apple or pear trees providing shade while adding structure to your garden's design. They

CHAPTER 5

stand as living sculptures, their branches painting the sky with blossoms in spring and heavy with fruit come late summer. Not only do they offer tasty treats, but they also create a dynamic focal point in any landscape.

Incorporating edible plants into your ornamental beds might sound tricky, but it's simpler than you think. Take those vibrant marigolds you've planted—now imagine them nestled alongside rich, earthy greens like kale or chard. The marigolds do double duty by adding splashes of color and deterring pests naturally. Herbs like rosemary and thyme weave through your flower beds, their fragrance mingling with the blooms while providing fresh seasonings just a few steps away from your kitchen. It's a garden that feeds both body and soul.

Designing such a harmonious blend requires a keen eye for both beauty and utility. Think of your garden as a layered tapestry where each plant plays a role. Tall fruit trees form the canopy, creating dappled sunlight for the shrubs and ground covers below. Use colorful and textured edible plants like rainbow Swiss chard or purple basil to add intrigue. Their vibrant shades contrast against the greens, making them pop visually while serving up flavor and nutrition. Layering plants this way maximizes space and boosts productivity, letting you harvest from different levels throughout the growing season.

Let's discuss some delightful plant pairings that perfectly balance aesthetics and growth. Imagine lavender's soft purple hues alongside blueberry bushes, creating a fragrant border buzzing with pollinators. The combination looks stunning and makes good use of space, as both thrive under similar conditions. Another clever duo involves kale interplanted with marigolds. The bright marigold blooms deter pests, allowing kale to flourish without interference, while their colors create a cheerful mosaic in the garden.

Maintaining an edible landscape involves more than just watering and weeding. Pruning becomes an art form here, balancing keeping plants healthy and ensuring they remain productive. Regularly trim fruit trees to promote airflow and sunlight penetration, which helps prevent disease while encouraging larger yields. Similarly, herbs benefit from regular harvesting, which keeps them bushy and prevents them from becoming leggy or woody.

Crop rotation is another key strategy for keeping your soil in peak condition. Changing plant locations each season prevents nutrient depletion and disrupts pest life cycles. This approach keeps the soil rich and plants thriving year after year, ensuring your edible landscape remains lush and productive.

Planning your harvests strategically can also enhance your garden's beauty and bounty. Stagger planting times so that while one crop matures, another is just beginning its journey. This technique, known as succession planting, keeps your garden vibrant and ensures a continuous supply of fresh produce throughout the season.

Another tip for maintaining such a garden is creating pathways inviting exploration. Use stepping stones or gravel paths to guide visitors through the garden, offering glimpses of hidden treasures tucked among the foliage. These paths provide access for maintenance and encourage you to engage with your garden daily, noticing subtle changes and savoring each new bloom or ripening fruit.

Finally, remember that an edible landscape is as much about personal expression as it is about function. Choose plants that reflect your tastes and preferences, both culinary and aesthetic. You may have a penchant for Mediterranean flavors; consider incorporating olive trees or grapevines into your design. Or you may be drawn to tropical vibes; banana plants or citrus trees could add that exotic touch while producing juicy delights.

Creating an edible landscape transforms gardening into an interactive experience that rewards all senses. Each visit becomes an opportunity to see the beauty unfold while savoring nature's offerings firsthand. It's not just about cultivating plants; it's about cultivating joy through thoughtful design that nourishes mind, body, and spirit alike. Your garden becomes more than just a pretty face. It's a vibrant tapestry woven from flavors, colors, textures, scents, and, most importantly, memories shared over meals with friends and family amidst its bountiful embrace.

Edible landscaping invites you to explore possibilities beyond traditional gardening boundaries. It is a creative endeavor where practicality meets artistry in every leaf and petal.

Themed Gardens: Creating a Cohesive Aesthetic

Have you ever wandered into a garden that felt like stepping into another world, where every element seemed to whisper tales and stir the imagination? This is the enchanting magic of themed gardens. They have the special power to transform ordinary spaces into genuinely immersive experiences, each with an astonishingly unique story to tell. Imagine crafting a fairy tale-inspired garden where whimsical elements like tiny cottages and enchanted pathways beckon visitors into a land of fantasy and enchantment. Gnarled trees adorned with lanterns dangling from their branches might light the way, casting a soft glow that dances across beds of colorful blooms, creating an atmosphere straight out of a storybook. The air, infused with the sweet scent of nostalgia and wonder, invites young and old alike to pause and linger a little longer, savoring the ethereal beauty.

Consider a Zen garden if tranquility is your goal and the need for a peaceful retreat draws you in. Pure and simplicity reign supreme here, and each stone and plant is placed deliberately. Raked gravel patterns mimic the gentle ripples of water, symbolizing serenity, while neatly trimmed bonsai trees offer a sense of calm and order. The garden becomes a sanctuary for reflection, a hallowed place where the mind can find peace amid the chaos of everyday life—a Zen escape from the ordinary. It's about stripping back the complexities to uncover the essentials, allowing nature's beauty to shine through in its purest and most harmonious form.

Planning and executing a themed garden involves a creative blend of artistry and practicality. Start by choosing plants and materials that align seamlessly with your vision. Fairy tale gardens might feature vibrant flowers like foxgloves and delphiniums, their tall, majestic spires adding vertical interest

CHAPTER 5

and bursts of vivid color. Consider incorporating decor that enhances the theme—perhaps a weathered wrought iron bench with intricate designs or a minor, gently burbling water feature that babbles softly in the background, drawing onlookers into its soothing melody. Zen gardens, on the other hand, benefit immensely from minimalism, drawing inspiration from Japanese traditions. Opt for evergreens and mosses that provide serene year-round beauty without demanding much attention, maintaining tranquility with ease.

Themes can vary widely, catering to a dizzying array of tastes and preferences. A Mediterranean garden brings the warmth of sun-drenched coastal landscapes to your backyard. Olive trees provide pleasant shade, while terracotta pots filled with aromatic herbs like rosemary and thyme add fragrance, evoking cherished memories of the Mediterranean. Stone walls and gravel paths complete this idyllic picture, evoking images of quaint, rustic villages perched on hillsides overlooking azure seas. Meanwhile, cottage gardens are all about abundance and charm, embracing a sense of playful whimsy. Picture overflowing borders filled with hollyhocks and lupines, their cheerful colors creating a riotous display against quaint wooden fences, a timeless tableau that bursts with life.

Achieving cohesion in themed gardens requires careful attention to the art of balance. Consistency in color palettes and textures helps create a unified and harmonious look that ties everything together seamlessly. Imagine using soft pastels for a fairy tale garden, where gentle hues of pink, purple, and blues blend harmoniously as if woven into a dream. In contrast, bold hues might dominate a tropical paradise theme, where vibrant reds and oranges catch the eye at every turn, commanding attention with their vivid allure. Harmony between hardscape and softscape elements is also crucial. Thought-provoking paths should lead seamlessly from one enchanting area to another, guiding visitors through your meticulously crafted narrative.

The key to success is steadfastly focusing on your theme throughout the design process. Avoid cluttering the space with unrelated elements that might disrupt the overall aesthetic and the story you're telling. Instead, let each component contribute meaningfully to the narrative, choosing elements that enhance and complement the vision. This might mean gently editing out certain plants or features that don't quite fit, ensuring that every piece contributes to the cohesive whole.

Themed gardens invite you to think outside the box and deeply inject your personality and imagination into your outdoor space. They offer endless possibilities for creativity and exploration and an opportunity to express yourself vividly through nature's versatile canvas. Whether you transport visitors to far-off lands or create intimate, cherished retreats closer to home, these gardens are reflections of your imagination made tangible, a living testament to your vision.

As we wrap up our exploration of creative gardening approaches in this enthralling chapter, remember that each technique offers unique opportunities to transform your green space into something truly special and memorable. From the intricate artistry of succulent gardens to the immersive worlds of themed gardens, every idea adds yet another layer of depth and richness to your outdoor haven, leaving an indelible mark on those who experience it.

In our next chapter, we'll delve with great anticipation into the world of sustainable gardening practices because what's better than a breathtakingly beautiful garden? One that's kind to the planet as well! We'll cover everything from ingenious water-wise strategies to organic methods that nurture both plants and the environment, ensuring ecological harmony. So stay tuned as we journey deeper into gardens that captivate our senses and leave a positive, lasting imprint on this wonderful world we all share.

THE GARDEN GUIDE "FUN FACTS FOR BUDDING GREEN THUMB'S"

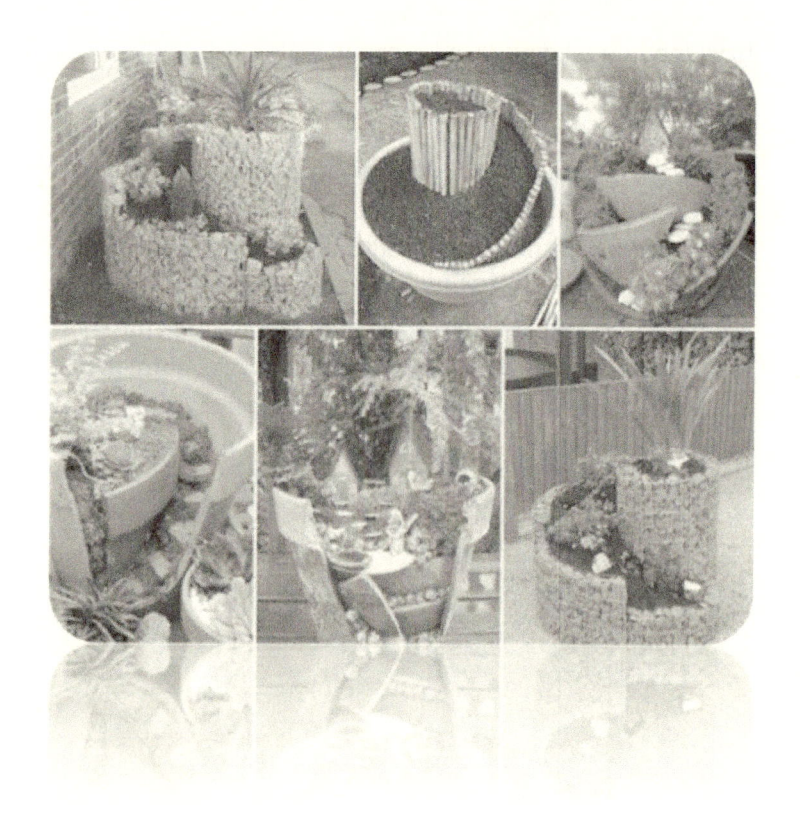

Chapter 6

Problem-Solving and Practical Tip

Troubleshooting Troubles: Solving Common Plant Problems

Ever find yourself staring at your garden, wondering why your once-thriving plants look more like they're auditioning for a role in a botanical horror movie? Fear not, because decoding plant distress is easier than you might think. Imagine being a plant detective, armed with a magnifying glass and a keen eye, ready to solve the mystery of the wilting leaves.

Plants communicate their woes through signs if you know where to look. Yellowing leaves are often the first red flag. They can signal all sorts of issues, from overwatering to nutrient deficiencies. Think of yellow leaves as your plant's way of waving a distress flag. But don't worry, it's not always dire. Sometimes, it's just a subtle hint that they need more love, perhaps a splash of fertilizer or a touch less water.

Wilting is another common cry for help. Picture leaves drooping as if they're too weary to face another day. This can be a sign of underwatering, but it could also indicate root rot from too much water. It's like the Goldilocks dilemma: your plant needs just the right amount of moisture. Checking the soil moisture with your finger can reveal whether your plant is parched or drowning.

When plants start looking poorly, it's time to play doctor and diagnose the ailment. Root rot and nutrient deficiencies are common culprits. Root rot is like a stealthy villain, creeping in with poor drainage. Dig gently around the roots; if they're mushy and dark, there's your answer. On the other hand, pale leaves suggest your plants might be hungry for nutrients. A soil test can help you determine what's lacking and guide your next steps.

Distinguishing between fungal and bacterial infections requires more sleuthing. Fungal infections often leave powdery or rusty marks on leaves, while bacterial issues can cause wet, oozy spots. Think of fungal problems as the mildew that shows up uninvited, while bacteria are the unwelcome guests that leave a mess. Treatment with appropriate fungicides or bactericides can mitigate the issue before it spreads like gossip at a garden club meeting.

Once you've identified the issue, let's discuss solutions and prevention strategies. Adjusting soil pH is a fantastic way to improve nutrient uptake; it's like giving your plants a balanced diet. Based on your soil test results (Cooperative Extension: Garden and Yard), use lime to raise pH or sulfur to lower it. Regular pruning promotes air circulation and keeps plants from becoming overly cozy with their neighbors. Imagine each snip as a breath of fresh air for your garden.

Proactive plant care is your secret weapon. Schedule regular health inspections like you would for a beloved pet. Look for any signs of distress before they become full-blown crises. Keeping a garden journal is another nifty trick. Note any issues and solutions; it's like creating your gardening encyclopedia (Chadwick). Plus, it's satisfying to look back and see how far you've come.

Interactive Element: Garden Detective Checklist

- **Yellow Leaves:** Check for overwatering or nutrient deficiency.
- **Wilting:** Assess soil moisture levels.
- **Root Health:** Inspect for signs of rot.
- **Leaf Spots:** Differentiate between fungal and bacterial.
- **Pruning Needs:** Identify areas needing better air circulation.
- **Soil pH:** Adjust for optimal nutrient absorption (Extension Gardener).

A proactive approach keeps your plants happy and thriving; no one likes an unhappy garden! Regular checkups prevent minor issues from snowballing into major ones. So channel your inner Sherlock Holmes and become the detective your garden needs!

Pest Patrol: Natural Solutions for Garden Invaders

Imagine a garden as a little kingdom, each plant a noble subject needing protection from marauding pests. Rather than reaching for chemical weaponry, consider eco-friendly alternatives that maintain the delicate balance of nature. Companion planting is a nifty trick to deter unwanted guests. Think of marigolds as bodyguards for your tomatoes, sending nematodes packing with their pungent odor. Basil can confuse aphids with their aromatic presence when nestled beside your tomatoes. These natural alliances create a harmonious environment where pests think twice before crashing the party.

For those who enjoy a bit of DIY, homemade insecticidal soap offers an effective solution. A simple mix of water, dish soap, and oil creates a potent spray that suffocates soft-bodied insects like aphids without harming beneficial critters. Imagine yourself as a garden alchemist, concocting protective potions that leave your plants safe and sound. This approach keeps your garden chemical-free while letting you play a hands-on role in your garden's defenses.

Recognizing common garden pests is crucial to effective management. Aphids are the garden's version of tiny vampires, sucking the life from tender new shoots. Look for clusters of these small green or black insects on the undersides of leaves. Their presence can lead to distorted growth and sticky honeydew deposits that attract ants. In contrast, snails and slugs are the slow-moving villains, leaving behind shiny trails and holes in leaves. Spotting these slimy intruders is easier under damp conditions when they're most active.

Managing these pests requires vigilance and a few clever tricks. Physical barriers like cloches and nets offer a simple yet effective defense by keeping pests at bay, allowing light and rain

CHAPTER 6

to reach your plants. Picture these as tiny fortresses guarding your treasured blooms. For more specific pests, pheromone traps can be a game-changer. They lure insects like moths with irresistible scents, reducing populations without chemicals. It's the garden equivalent of setting out bait for unwelcome critters.

Creating a biodiverse environment is one of the best defenses against pests. By welcoming beneficial insects like ladybugs, you introduce natural predators that happily munch on aphids and other pesky invaders. Planting a variety of species also helps deter monocultures that invite pest infestations. A mix of flowering plants attracts pollinators and beneficial insects, creating a bustling ecosystem of allies ready to defend your garden's honor.

As you cultivate this balanced ecosystem, you'll notice that pests become less of an issue over time. Encourage ladybugs by planting dill or fennel; consider these as VIP seating for your garden's beneficial insects. These tiny allies play a significant role in keeping pest populations in check, transforming your garden into a self-sustaining haven.

Incorporating diverse plantings ensures that no single pest can devastate your garden. Mix herbs with flowers and vegetables to create visual interest and natural pest deterrents. This diversity confuses pests and reduces the risk of widespread infestations. It's like hosting a lively garden party where everyone gets along, except for the gate-crashing pests who find themselves outnumbered and unwelcome.

Creating such a well-balanced ecosystem requires patience and observation, but it pays off in healthier plants and fewer chemical interventions. As you spend more time among your plants, you'll develop a keen sense of spotting potential issues early on. This proactive approach allows you to address problems swiftly, keeping your garden vibrant and thriving.

Visual Element: Pest Identification Chart

- **Aphids:** Small green or black insects on leaf undersides.
- **Snails/Slugs:** Slimy trails and leaf holes.
- **Ladybugs:** Red with black spots; beneficial insect.
- **Cloches/Nets:** Physical barriers for pest protection.
- **Pheromone Traps:** Lure specific insect pests.

This holistic approach emphasizes nature's interconnectedness, encouraging you to work with it rather than against it. By fostering an environment that supports beneficial insects and diversifies plantings, you'll find yourself engaging in an ongoing dialogue with your garden. This conversation shapes each season's growth and beauty.

CHAPTER 6

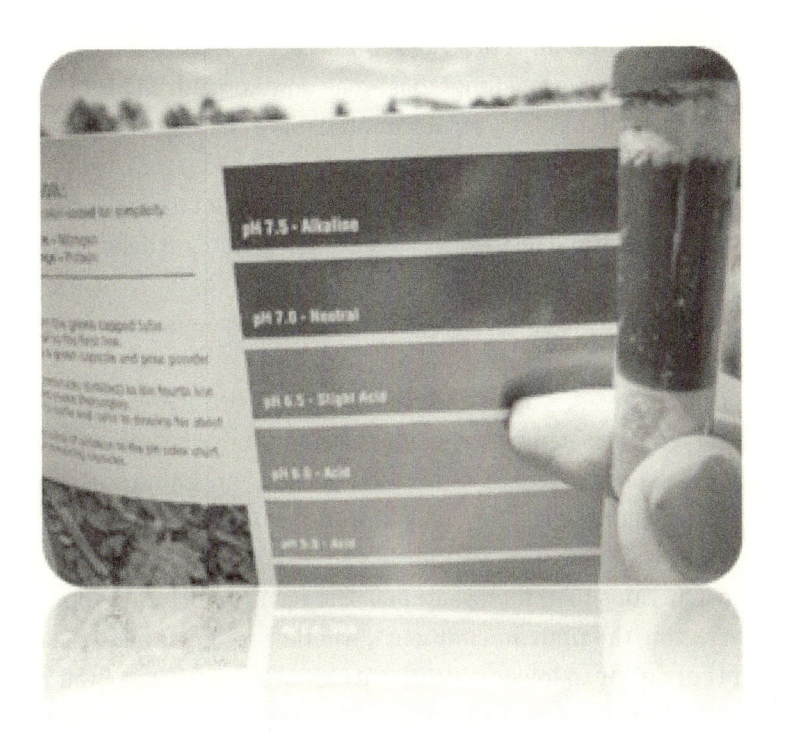

Soil Secrets: Optimizing Conditions for Plant Growth

Healthy soil is like a five-star hotel for your plants, offering all the comforts they need to flourish. The secret sauce lies in its structure and the vibrant community of microorganisms bustling beneath the surface. Organic matter is your soil's best friend. It keeps the soil loose and airy, making it easier for roots to spread and breathe. Think of it as adding fluff to a pillow to provide more comfort for your plants. Organic matter acts like a sponge, soaking up water and holding onto nutrients, ensuring your plants aren't thirsty or hungry.

But that's not all. A diverse soil microbiome teems with life, hosting bacteria and fungi that break down organic matter into nutrients your plants can absorb. It's like a bustling downtown market, where everything is constantly traded and transformed. These tiny organisms create a lively ecosystem that supports plant growth and resilience. They even help ward off diseases by outcompeting harmful pathogens for resources. So, a healthy microbiome is like having a security team in your soil, keeping the bad guys at bay.

Soil testing is a must to get your soil in tip-top shape. Think of it as a health checkup for your garden. At-home soil test kits are handy tools for analyzing your soil's pH and nutrient levels. Grab one from your local garden center, and follow the instructions to gather a sample. The results will guide you in selecting the right amendments, whether adding lime to raise pH or sulfur to lower it. With this knowledge, you can tailor your soil to meet your plants' needs. Amendments like compost or well-rotted manure are significant for enriching the soil. They're like superfoods for your garden, packed with nutrients that feed both plants and the soil's microbial life.

Understanding soil types can feel like reading a book in a foreign language, but it's worth the effort. Clay soil can be stubborn, holding onto water and nutrients with a vice-like grip. It's heavy and often compacts easily, making it challenging for roots to break through. But don't despair! Mixing in organic matter can improve drainage and loosen up the structure, giving roots room to breathe. Sandy soil is the opposite; it drains too quickly, leaving plants parched. Adding organic matter here helps retain moisture and nutrients, creating a more balanced environment.

Keeping the soil healthy over time requires some clever strategies. Crop rotation is an oldie but a goodie. By alternating the types of plants grown in an area each year, you prevent nutrient depletion and break pest cycles. It's like moving furniture around to freshen up a room and keep things interesting and balanced. Mulching is another fantastic practice that protects against erosion and nutrient loss. A good layer of mulch acts like a warm blanket in winter and a sunshade in summer. It conserves moisture, suppresses weeds, and gradually breaks down to feed the soil.

Long-term soil health doesn't happen overnight, but consistent care makes it the foundation of a thriving garden. Just like you wouldn't skip regular meals or exercise for yourself, your garden needs ongoing attention to stay strong and productive. Regularly amending the soil with compost and practicing techniques like crop rotation keep it fertile and vibrant year after year.

With these insights at your fingertips, you can nurture soil supporting robust plant growth. Embrace these strategies as part of your gardening routine, and watch your plants respond with vitality and vigor. The rewards are worth every bit of effort you invest. So, dig into your soil, not literally, and discover the secrets that turn ordinary dirt into extraordinary growing ground.

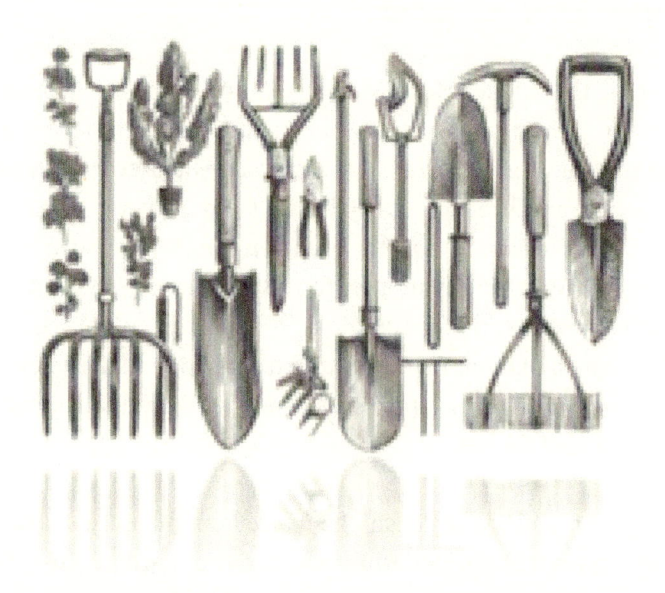

Efficient Gardening Tools: Making Your Job Easier

Imagine stepping into your garden armed with the best tools that seem almost magical in their ability to make tasks easier. Ergonomic hand tools are game-changers designed to reduce the strain on your wrists and hands as you dig, plant, and prune. These tools fit comfortably in your grip, letting you work longer without feeling like you've wrestled a bear by the end of the day. Look for tools with padded handles and a design that aligns with the natural movement of your wrist.

Now, let's talk about those trusty garden carts and wheelbarrows. These are like having a reliable sidekick ready to haul anything from soil to freshly picked produce. Opt for a multi-

CHAPTER 6

purpose cart that can transform from a flatbed to a wheelbarrow with a simple adjustment. It's like having a Swiss Army knife on wheels, saving you trips back and forth and giving your back a break from heavy lifting.

Selecting the right tool for the job makes all the difference. When it comes to pruners, choosing the right type depends on what you're snipping. Bypass pruners work best for live plants, slicing cleanly without crushing stems. Anvil pruners, with one straight and one curved blade, are better suited for dry, brittle branches. It's like having a fine dining knife set; each one has a specific purpose that makes life easier.

Hoes and cultivators are indispensable for soil preparation. A sturdy hoe can clear weeds and break up soil clumps in one fell swoop. Meanwhile, a cultivator with its curved tines helps aerate the soil, mixing nutrients to create a welcoming environment for seeds. Think of these tools as the prep chefs of your garden, ensuring everything's ready for planting.

Once you've invested in quality tools, maintaining them is key to keeping them in top shape. Cleaning is crucial; wash the dirt off after each use and dry them thoroughly. Sharpen blades regularly to ensure they cut efficiently. It's like keeping your kitchen knives sharp; it makes every task smoother and safer. Proper storage prevents rust and damage. Please keep them in a dry place, perhaps hanging on a pegboard or in a dedicated shed space.

Technology has entered the gardening world with gadgets that make life even easier. Battery-powered tillers and weeders zip through tasks without needing gas or muscle power. They're lightweight yet powerful, tackling weeds and tilling soil like mini garden superheroes. For watering, intelligent irrigation systems equipped with sensors adjust watering schedules based on soil moisture levels and weather forecasts. It's like having a personal assistant for your garden, ensuring plants receive just the right amount of care.

Smart Tool Selection Chart

- **Ergonomic Hand Tools:** For comfort and reduced strain.
- **Multi-purpose Carts:** Versatile hauling solutions.
- **Bypass Pruners:** Ideal for live plants.
- **Anvil Pruners:** Perfect for dry branches.
- **Battery-Powered Tillers:** Lightweight soil preparation.
- **Smart Irrigation Systems:** Automated watering efficiency.

Innovative tools don't just save time; they enhance your gardening experience, leaving you with more energy to enjoy your green space. With the right tools, gardening becomes less of a chore and more of a joy-filled adventure, where every task is an opportunity to connect with nature. Embrace these modern marvels and watch how they transform your gardening routine into something special.

Weathering the Storm: Protecting Your Plants from the Elements

Weather can be a gardener's best friend or worst enemy, and sometimes it feels like your plants are at the mercy of Mother Nature's whims. Frost has a way of sneaking in overnight, leav-

CHAPTER 6

ing your tender sprouts looking like they've had an unfortunate run-in with Mr. Freeze. Frost can damage plant cells, causing leaves to wilt or turn black like a bad sunburn. To mitigate frost damage, consider covering your plants with bed sheets, burlap, or specially designed-frost cloths. These coverings act like cozy blankets, trapping heat close to the ground and keeping those chilly fingers of frost at bay. Early risers can also spray water on frost-covered plants in the morning, helping them thaw gently and preventing further damage.

On the other hand, heatwaves can turn your garden into a sauna. The relentless sun bakes the soil, evaporates moisture faster than you can say "sunburn," and leaves plants gasping for a breath of cool air. In these scorching times, hydration is key. Water plants deeply in the early morning or late evening to minimize evaporation. Mulching is a lifesaver, acting like a sunhat for your soil, conserving moisture, and keeping roots cool. For added relief, strategically place shade cloths or umbrellas to shield vulnerable plants from the intense midday sun. It's like setting up beach umbrellas for your leafy friends without the piña coladas.

Preparing for extreme weather is all about having a plan. Windbreaks, such as fences or hedges, can protect plants from harsh winds that threaten to flatten your prized dahlias. Picture them as bodyguards standing firm against gusty assaults. Row covers and cloches provide another layer of defense, insulating plants against both frost and wind. They're like tiny greenhouses, offering protection while letting sunlight and rain reach plants.

Microclimates are the secret weapon of savvy gardeners. Understanding and manipulating these localized climate variations allows you to create protective havens within your garden. Walls and fences can absorb heat during the day and release it at night, providing warmth to nearby plants, like giving them a heated blanket on a chilly night. Meanwhile, planting taller vegetation on the sunny side creates natural shade zones where more delicate plants can thrive away from direct heat.

After a storm passes, it's time to assess and assist your plants' recovery. Damaged branches should be pruned back to healthy growth to prevent disease entry points and encourage new growth. It's like giving your plants a haircut after a rough patch—they'll look better and feel rejuvenated. Following severe weather, replenishing soil nutrients becomes crucial. Adding organic matter like compost or well-rotted manure revitalizes the soil, providing essential nutrients to help plants bounce back.

Recovery isn't just about physical repairs; it's also about nurturing resilience. Watering deeply helps wash away salts that might have accumulated during heavy rains or drought conditions. Ensure your garden has adequate drainage to prevent waterlogging during rainy spells; raised beds or adding sand to heavy clay soils can improve drainage efficiency.

Incorporating these strategies safeguards your plants and builds a garden that can adapt to changing conditions with grace and vigor. By anticipating weather challenges and employing protective measures, you'll find that your garden becomes more robust and less susceptible to the whims of fluctuating climates.

CHAPTER 6

Gardening with an eye on weather conditions fosters a deeper connection with the environment, a reminder of nature's cycles, and the need for flexibility and innovation in our growing practices. As you implement these strategies, you'll develop intuition for anticipating weather shifts and preparing accordingly. Plus, there's a certain satisfaction in knowing you've outsmarted Mother Nature just enough to keep your garden thriving through all her tests.

The joy of gardening lies in this dance with nature, balancing protection with adaptation, learning from each season's trials, and celebrating triumphs big and small with every new blossom or leaf unfurled in defiance of adversity.

Smart Watering: Techniques for Optimal Hydration

Watering plants isn't as simple as it seems; just water over the plant, and voila, you're done! However, there's an intricate art to it that, when mastered, differentiates between a thriving garden and one that's struggling. Each plant is unique in its hydration needs, akin to the diverse preferences of individuals, each liking their tea at just the right temperature. Overwatering can be as detrimental as neglect, leading to the ominous threat of root rot. This insidious deterioration is concealed beneath the pristine surface, where roots become wet mush incapable of facilitating essential nutrient uptake. It's comparable to over-soaking a sponge, rendering it heavy, unusable, and inefficient. Conversely, letting plants dry out to the extreme leaves them literally gasping for a revitalizing drink. At this point, their leaves droop sorrowfully, their edges crisp up in protest, and they adopt an overall appearance reflective of being scorched under an unforgiving sun. Recognizing these symptoms is crucial, enabling you to adjust your watering routine accordingly to maintain the joy and vigor in your plant companions.

To conquer the intricacies of watering, one must adopt efficient techniques that utilize water judiciously while transforming your garden into a verdant paradise. For example, drip irrigation systems are the epitome of precision gardening, much like having a personal assistant for your green companions, delivering hydration directly to the roots where it's most needed. This innovative approach cuts down on excessive water usage and reduces evaporation and waste significantly, making each drop truly count. For optimal efficiency, setting timers to water early in the morning or during the calm of late afternoon is advised. During these cooler parts of the day, evaporation is minimized, ensuring your plants receive the maximum benefit from the water they are given.

Embrace the wonders of the modern age with technology as your ally in the quest for optimal hydration! Utilize soil moisture sensors, the small yet ingenious devices that fundamentally transform the guessing game of watering into a science. They diligently measure moisture levels in the soil, alerting you precisely when your plants require a refill of nature's tonic, akin to having a knowledgeable garden whisperer at your disposal. Additionally, rainwater harvesting systems are another strategic asset, enabling you to collect rainwater in barrels, efficiently stockpiling this free bounty of nature for future use. Such systems appeal to environmentally conscious gardeners aiming to reduce their environmental footprint while nurturing their verdant oasis.

Water conservation transcends merely limiting usage; it's about employing water more intelligently. Consider mulching, the unsung hero in the conservation narrative. This practice entails spreading a generous layer of organic material, such as straw or wood chips, over the soil. Mulch acts as a formidable barrier against moisture evaporation, akin to a snug blanket preserving the warmth and moisture, prolonging soil moistness considerably. Pair this with cultivating drought-tolerant species, which inherently require substantially less hydration, and you've successfully crafted a winning strategy for a sustainable garden.

The Beauty of Resilient Plant Selections

Opting for plants that can withstand a bit of thirst is a wise decision, especially when cultivating in hot or particularly arid climates. Succulents, along with other native species, have evolved specialized mechanisms to thrive on minimal hydration, rendering them low-maintenance selections for diligent yet busy gardeners. These hardy, adaptive plants conserve precious water resources and contribute unique textures and vibrant colors, enriching your garden's overall aesthetic appeal.

By incorporating these watering strategies and embracing available technologies, you create a visually striking and brilliantly efficient garden. Proper watering is the cornerstone of fostering healthier roots, more vigorous plants, and dazzling blooms. It conserves time and resources, granting you the liberty to savor more of the joys that gardening offers without the perpetual stress associated with maintenance.

In closing this chapter, we reiterate that a well-watered garden epitomizes a joyful garden. It's about achieving that delightful equilibrium where plants flourish bountifully without squandering resources. Equipped with these strategies in your gardening arsenal, you're well-prepared to tackle hydration challenges with confidence and zest. As we venture onward, consider how these practices integrate holistically into your garden's ecosystem. In the upcoming chapter, we will delve into imaginative methods to infuse your garden space with artistic flair, transforming it into not merely a sphere of growth but also a dynamic canvas for creative expression and innovative endeavors.

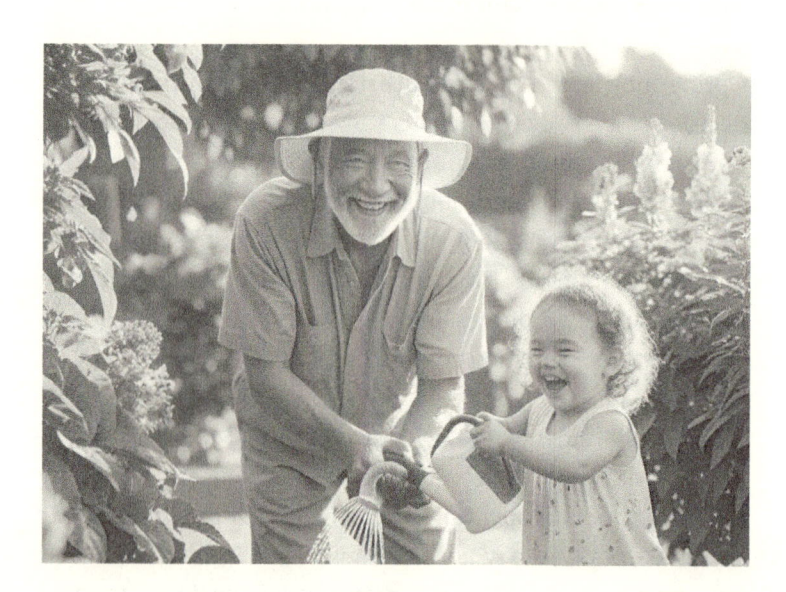

Chapter 7

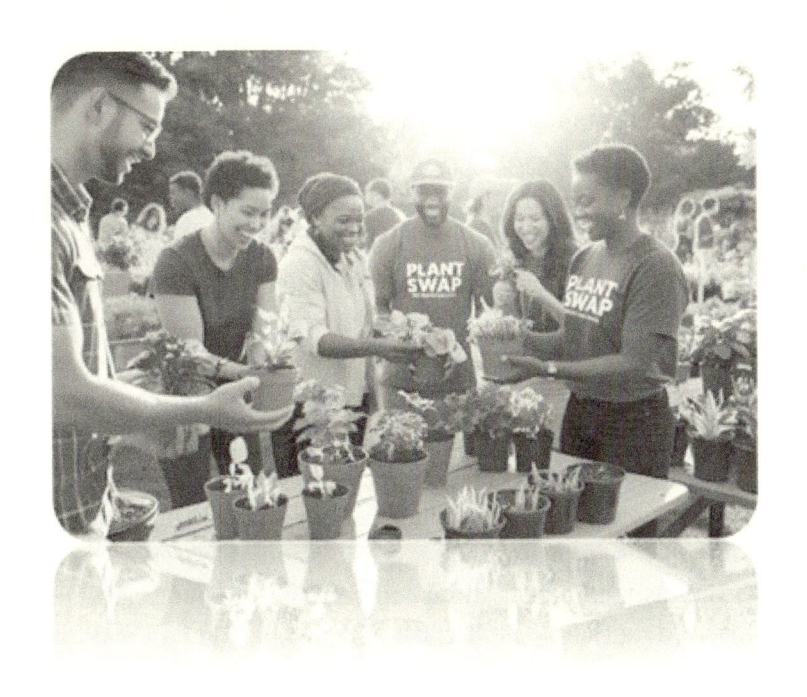

Gardening with Community and Connection

Plant Swaps and Shares: Building Community Through Gardening

Picture this: a bustling community hall filled with people exchanging smiles and potted treasures. Each plant has a story, and every gardener is eager to share theirs. Welcome to the world of plant swaps, where the currency is green, leafy, and sometimes spiky. These events are more than just a chance to score a new fern or succulent. They're vibrant gatherings that foster community spirit and promote biodiversity. Plant swaps encourage gardeners to diversify their collections while learning from each other's experiences. Imagine the joy of swapping your propagated spider plant for a new variety of basil, expanding your green repertoire while making a new friend.

Local plant swap events are like the social butterflies of the gardening world, flitting about and spreading joy. They draw people out of their homes and into shared spaces, nurturing connections as much as they do plants. Hosting a successful plant swap requires a little planning but promises big rewards. First, choose a venue that's accessible and roomy enough for enthusiastic exchanges; think community centers or local parks. Pick a date that doesn't clash with major holidays or local events, ensuring maximum participation. Promote the event through social media, community boards, and word of mouth. Creating an inviting atmosphere will attract both seasoned gardeners and curious newcomers alike.

There's something magical about sharing plants. It's not just

CHAPTER 7

about watching your collection grow without emptying your wallet. It's about strengthening community bonds through shared gardening experiences. When you share cuttings or seeds with others, you're not just passing on plants; you're sharing knowledge, hope, and the promise of growth. Every plant you exchange carries a piece of your garden's story, creating a living tapestry woven from countless origins.

Joining local and online plant swaps expands these opportunities even further. Whether you're exchanging seeds with a neighbor or trading cuttings with someone across the globe through a Facebook group, each swap enriches your gardening journey. Online swaps provide access to rare varieties that might not be available locally, while community-driven events offer face-to-face interactions and the chance to meet fellow enthusiasts. Consider joining forums where like-minded gardeners congregate to discuss their latest finds and share tips on successful swaps.

Interactive Element: Swap Success Checklist

Create a checklist for organizing or participating in a plant swap event to ensure everything runs smoothly and everyone leaves with a smile and maybe a new favorite plant! Include items such as:

- Gather pest-free plants or seeds for exchange.
- Label each plant with its name and care instructions.
- Bring containers or bags to transport new plants.
- Engage with other participants by sharing stories about your plants.

- Follow any established swap rules to ensure fairness and fun for all.

Plant swaps are more than just exchanges of greenery. They're celebrations of community and connection, proof that the love of gardening knows no bounds, geographical or otherwise. They remind us that our gardens are part of something larger, a shared passion that extends beyond borders and blooms in every corner of the world. So grab your favorite potted companion and head to the nearest swap. You might leave with more than just new plants; you could find new friends and stories to enrich your gardening life.

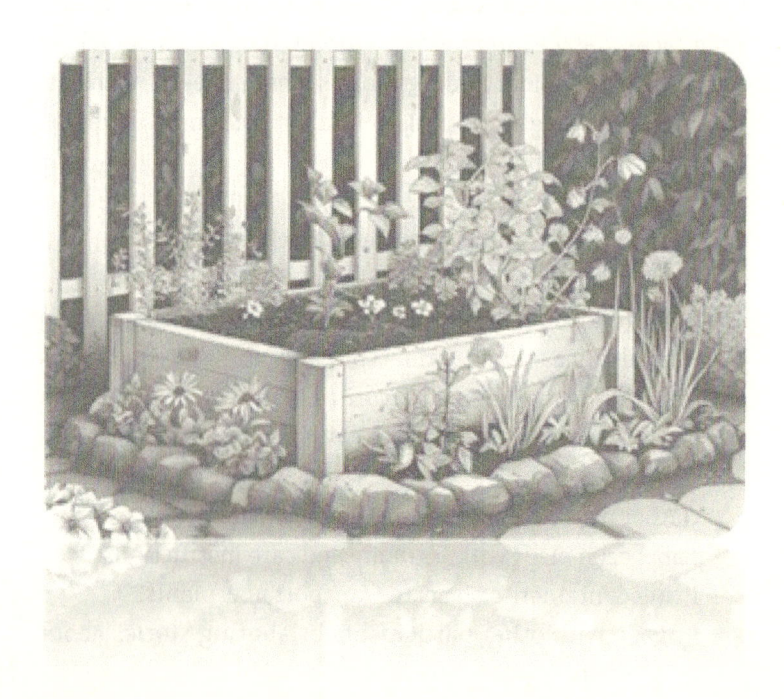

CHAPTER 7

Community Gardens: Cultivating Shared Spaces

Imagine a patch of green nestled in the heart of your neighborhood, where tomatoes ripen under the sun and neighbors gather, trowels in hand, to nurture both botanical and communal growth. This is the soul of a community garden. These shared spaces are like a breath of fresh air in urban landscapes, providing access to fresh produce, fostering social interaction, and promoting collaboration. Community gardens ensure that fresh vegetables aren't just a luxury in places where a supermarket might be a bus ride away. They improve food security by offering an accessible bounty of fruits and vegetables right where people live.

Community gardens are more than just plots of earth; they're vibrant hubs of connectivity and learning. Here, people of diverse backgrounds come together, sharing tips, stories, and seeds. These interactions cultivate not only plants but also friendships and understanding. In our fast-paced world, taking time to garden with others can slow down the rush, allowing for genuine connections over shared goals. It's like a team sport but with more photosynthesis and less sweating.

Joining or starting a community garden can be a transformative experience. Begin by researching existing initiatives around you. Many cities have networks of community gardens, often managed by local councils or nonprofit organizations. Reach out to them to learn about available plots or waiting lists. If you're inspired to start a new community garden, gather a group of like-minded individuals and start the conversation. Securing land might seem daunting, but consider underused spaces like vacant lots or rooftops. You'll need to assess soil quality and water access, but the effort pays off with a flourishing garden.

Successful community gardens dot cities across the globe, each telling its own story. Urban rooftop gardens are sprouting up in metropolises, contributing to local food networks and reducing urban heat islands. Imagine tomatoes growing against a backdrop of skyscrapers! School-based gardens also play a pivotal role in education, turning science lessons into hands-on experiences. Students learn about ecosystems, sustainability, and nutrition as they watch their efforts blossom into tangible results.

Yet, like any group endeavor, community gardening comes with its fair share of challenges. Coordinating volunteer efforts can feel enthusiastic but not always predictable, like herding cats. To combat this, establish a clear schedule that accommodates different availability. Regular meetings help keep everyone on the same page and maintain momentum. Managing resources and funding requires creativity and persistence. Local businesses might sponsor tools or supplies in exchange for good PR; think of it as a win-win situation.

Funding can also be a hurdle. Look into grants available for community projects or crowdfunding platforms where you can rally support. Every little bit helps when it comes to buying seeds or improving infrastructure, like installing rain barrels for sustainable watering solutions. Creative problem-solving is your best tool here; think outside the planter box!

CHAPTER 7

A thriving community garden is both a triumph and a testament to what people can achieve together. They beautify neighborhoods, reduce carbon footprints, and nurture both the earth and human spirit. As you walk through rows of thriving plants, know that you're part of something bigger—a movement towards sustainable living and stronger communities.

Community gardens stand as living testaments to shared efforts and collective joys. They prove that when people join forces with nature—and each other, the results are bountiful beyond measure. They remind us that in every seed planted lies potential for growth and connection, resilience, and hope in our collective future.

These spaces offer much more than produce; they cultivate resilience and foster unexpected friendships sprouting amidst rows of kale and sunflowers. When gardeners come together, they create more than lush landscapes; they build communities rooted in understanding and shared purpose, a garden of plants and people flourishing in harmony.

Hosting Garden Parties: Celebrating Your Green Achievements

Picture this: your lush and vibrant garden is the backdrop for a gathering of friends and family. The scent of blooming flowers wafts through the air as laughter and chatter mingle with birdsong. Hosting garden parties is a fantastic way to celebrate your gardening triumphs and share the fruits of your labor. It's not just about showing off your green thumb; it's an opportunity to create memorable experiences in a setting that reflects your hard work and passion.

Inviting guests for a tour of your garden is a lovely way to start the party. Guide them through the pathways you've carefully tended, showcasing seasonal blooms and the bounty of your harvest. Imagine the delight on their faces as they admire your prize-winning roses or sample fresh strawberries plucked straight from the vine. These moments transform simple admiration into shared joy, creating lasting memories for everyone involved.

Planning a garden party involves creativity and attention to detail. Start by selecting a theme that complements your garden's natural beauty. Whether you choose a whimsical fairy tale setting or a chic minimalist affair, coordinating decorations with your theme can elevate the atmosphere. Consider using natural elements like twinkling string lights or lanterns to add a magical touch as dusk falls. When it comes to food, opt for garden-friendly dishes that are easy to prepare and enjoy outdoors. Fresh salads, finger foods, and refreshing beverages infused with herbs from your garden keep things light and delicious.

Entertainment is key to engaging guests and ensuring the party is lively. Consider hosting gardening workshops or demonstrations as part of the festivities. Show off your composting skills or teach guests how to propagate plants; these activities provide both education and fun. If you'd rather keep things lighthearted, organize garden-themed games or quizzes. A scavenger hunt that encourages exploration around your garden can be a hit with both kids and adults.

CHAPTER 7

Garden parties aren't just about plants; they're about people. Gathering in a garden fosters connection and camaraderie, strengthening relationships through shared experiences. The informal setting encourages conversation and laughter, breaking down social barriers and allowing guests to relax and enjoy themselves. It's incredible how a simple gathering can spark meaningful gardening knowledge and tips exchanges. Before you know it, you'll find yourself learning as much as you're sharing, whether it's about pest control or creative landscaping ideas.

Hosting a garden party offers social benefits beyond the day's enjoyment. It provides a platform for exchanging gardening wisdom, with each guest bringing unique insights and experiences. These interactions enrich our understanding of gardening and open our minds to new possibilities. By celebrating our green achievements together, we cultivate our gardens and sense of community.

Picture yourself at the center of this vibrant scene, surrounded by people who appreciate the beauty of nature as much as you do. The garden acts as a canvas for connection and celebration, where each plant tells a story, and every flower adds its color to the tapestry of shared memories. As the sun sets and soft lighting illuminates the space, you'll feel a sense of fulfillment knowing that your garden has brought people together in such a meaningful way.

So grab those invitations, dust off your picnic blankets, and get ready to host a garden party that celebrates not only your achievements but also the joy of being part of a thriving gardening community. Whether it's an intimate gathering or a lively affair, these events remind us that gardens are more than just plots of land; they're spaces where friendships blossom, creativity flourishes, and life is celebrated in all its beautiful forms.

As you plan your next garden party, remember that the most essential element is the connection you foster with those who gather around you. Through shared laughter, learning, and celebration, you're not just showcasing your green thumb; you're cultivating relationships that will continue growing long after the party ends. So, raise a glass (or a watering can) to your achievements and enjoy the company of those who share your passion for gardening!

Garden Clubs and Groups: Finding Your Plant Tribe

Imagine a room buzzing with chatter, where everyone's eyes light up at the mention of a new fertilizer or a rare orchid. This is the magic of garden clubs, where plant enthusiasts gather to exchange stories, tips, and even seeds. These clubs are more than just meetings; they're communities of like-minded individuals who share a passion for all things green. Regular gatherings often focus on specific gardening topics, offering opportunities to learn from each other and collaborate on projects. Picture a session where you discuss composting techniques or the best plants for shade, all while sipping on a cup of tea surrounded by people who genuinely understand your love for the soil.

Joining a garden club is easier than you might think. Start

CHAPTER 7

by checking out community centers or local libraries. They often have bulletin boards brimming with information about clubs you can join. Online platforms also have treasure troves of gardening groups, with forums and social media pages dedicated to every niche interest you can imagine. If you're feeling adventurous and there isn't a club nearby, consider starting your own. Gather friends or fellow garden enthusiasts and set up regular meetups. Choose a cozy cafe or someone's garden as your meeting spot, and let the plant talk flow.

Being part of a gardening group comes with its perks. You'll have access to a wealth of shared resources and expertise to take your gardening game to the next level. Imagine borrowing specialized tools or sharing rare seeds that you wouldn't easily find elsewhere. These groups often organize group projects and initiatives, from beautifying a local park to setting up informational booths at community events. The sense of accomplishment from working together on these projects is unparalleled, like watching a flower you planted bloom for the first time.

Garden clubs are known for their creative activities and outings that keep members engaged and inspired. Group visits to botanical gardens and nurseries offer fresh perspectives and ideas for your own gardening endeavors. Imagine wandering through rows of exotic plants with fellow enthusiasts, snapping photos, and sharing tips on propagation. Some clubs organize collaborative community beautification projects, where members roll up their sleeves to transform neglected spaces into vibrant gardens. It's a hands-on way to give back to the community while bonding with others who share your passion.

One delightful anecdote comes from a garden club that decided to host an annual "Plant Lovers' Picnic." Each member brought dishes featuring ingredients from their gardens, such as salads with homegrown herbs and desserts adorned with edible flowers. They spent the day sharing gardening triumphs and challenges, exchanging tips on pest control, and admiring each other's green creations. These events foster friendships and connections that extend beyond the garden, creating a support network for life's ups and downs.

Participating in garden clubs isn't just about plants; it's about finding your tribe, a group of people who understand the thrill of spotting the first bud on a newly planted rose or the frustration of battling stubborn weeds. It's like being part of an exclusive club where everyone knows the secret handshake (it might involve soil under your fingernails). You'll find yourself swapping tales of gardening victories and commiserating over setbacks with people who genuinely get it.

So why not take the plunge? Whether you're an experienced gardener or just starting, there's a club out there waiting for you. These groups offer more than just gardening knowledge; they provide a sense of belonging and camaraderie that can enhance your life in countless ways. Plus, there's something special about knowing that whatever challenges your garden throws at you, there's a group of friends ready to offer advice, encouragement, and maybe a cutting or two. Your plant tribe is out there; all you have to do is reach out and join in on the fun!

CHAPTER 7

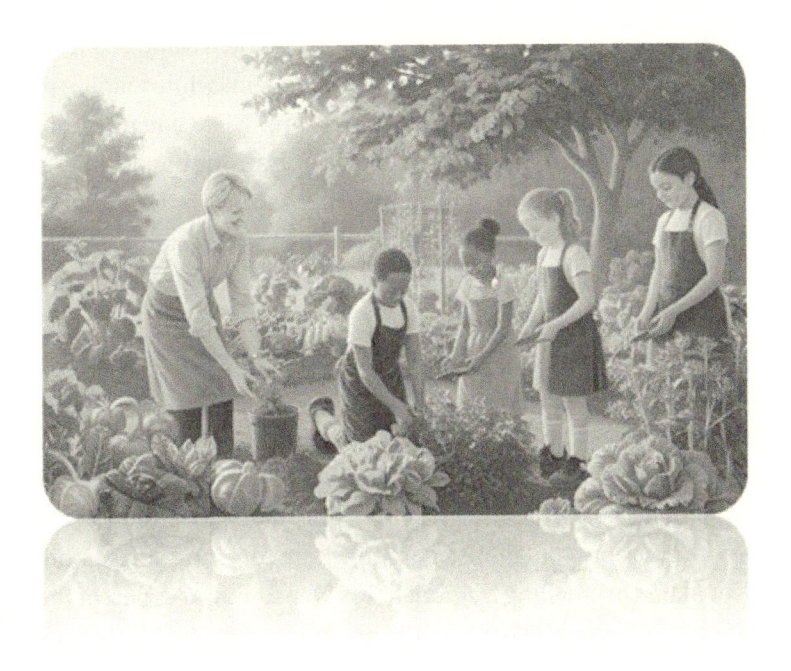

Educational Gardens: Teaching and Learning Together

Imagine a classroom without walls, where nature is the blackboard and every leaf, root, or bug has a lesson to teach. That's the magic of educational gardens. These spaces transform learning into an adventure, blending the sciences with the arts in a far more engaging setting than any textbook. Biology and ecology come alive in these gardens—not through diagrams or lectures but through hands-on encounters with the natural world. Kids (and adults, too!) get to see how plants grow, understand their role in ecosystems, and witness the delicate balance that sustains life.

Think about it: planting a seed teaches patience and observation. Watching it sprout shows how life begins while tending to it offers lessons in responsibility and care. When you integrate math and science, you unlock a world of learning opportunities. Measuring plots for planting involves geometry. Calculating soil needs or water requirements sharpens math skills. Believe it or not, planning the layout of a garden can involve more strategy than a chess game.

Creating an educational garden doesn't need to be complicated. Start by designing spaces that invite curiosity. Consider incorporating interpretive signs and labels that explain plant species and their roles in the ecosystem. Sensory gardens can add layers of interaction—imagine a garden where touching soft lamb's ear plants or smelling fragrant herbs is encouraged as part of the learning process. These tactile experiences make knowledge tangible, engaging learners in ways conventional settings can't.

The benefits of educational gardens are as varied as the plants they host. They encourage critical thinking as learners ask about growth patterns, pest behaviors, and weather impacts. Real-world applications bring classroom knowledge into focus, making concepts stick because they've been experienced firsthand. It's one thing to read about photosynthesis; it's another to see it in action as sunshine fuels the plants you've nurtured.

Success stories abound when it comes to educational gardens making a positive impact. School gardens are particularly effective at supporting STEM education. Picture students measuring plant growth rates for science projects or using data from their garden plots to create graphs in math class. These gardens turn abstract ideas into concrete knowledge. They give context to classroom lessons and help students see connections between subjects.

Community gardens also shine by offering workshops and classes that teach gardening skills while fostering community engagement. Imagine neighbors coming together for a Saturday workshop on composting led by someone who's been doing it in their own backyard for years. These gatherings provide a platform for sharing knowledge across generations and backgrounds.

Educational gardens are more than just learning tools; they are bridges connecting people with nature and each other. They invite exploration and discovery, sparking curiosity that transcends age or experience. Here, mistakes aren't failures; they're learning opportunities. A plant that doesn't thrive becomes a discussion point rather than a disappointment.

For those pondering how to start such a garden, begin small but think big. You could transform a section of your schoolyard or community center into a thriving hub of learning and growth. Engage local experts—from master gardeners to enthusiastic amateurs, who can contribute insights and guidance. Collaborate with educators who are willing to integrate garden activities into their curriculum.

Imagine a garden alive with students eagerly tending rows of vegetables or observing pollinators at work among native flowers. Picture them journaling about changes they observe over seasons, honing their writing skills while developing an appreciation for nature's cycles. Educational gardens offer more than academic enrichment; they nurture empathy by fostering connections between people and the planet.

These green spaces are classrooms without boundaries where learning happens organically (pun intended!). They offer lessons in sustainability and academics, teaching future generations how to care for our earth while reaping its rewards responsibly.

So why not grab your trowel and start planting seeds, not just of plants but of knowledge? Whether you're helping create an educational garden or simply enjoying one already established near you, remember this: every leaf has something to say if we're willing to listen closely enough. And in these vibrant classrooms, there's always room for one more eager learner ready to see what stories the soil has yet to share.

Online Gardening Communities: Connecting in the Digital Age

Imagine a world where your garden is not merely a secluded space reserved for solitude and tranquility but a vibrant part of an immense, interconnected tapestry of flourishing green spaces shared by individuals across the globe, united by a collective passion for nurturing nature. This is the transformative power of online gardening communities, which have remarkably bridged the gap for gardeners from all walks of life, whether they find themselves in the heart of bustling cities or the serene seclusion of the countryside. These dynamic

CHAPTER 7

platforms provide a sanctuary where individuals can exchange experiences, share invaluable tips, and forge lasting friendships over a shared, undying love for all things botanical. Popular gardening forums and social media groups function like bustling marketplaces teeming with diverse ideas and boundless inspiration. Esteemed websites such as GardenWeb or interactive forums like Permies have assembled a mosaic of individuals who, despite geographical discrepancies, find solidarity in their unyielding passion for cultivating life. Gardeners discover a profound sense of community within these virtual spaces, even while physically apart.

Engaging with these digital realms is an experience as seamless as sharing a snapshot of your most recent bloom or seeking guidance for a fern struggling in distress. Your smartphone transforms into a lens through which a global garden expedition unfolds before your eyes. Posting images of your cherished plant babies on platforms like Instagram or Facebook serves as a testament to your dedication and invites constructive feedback and heartfelt encouragement from fellow enthusiasts. By immersing yourself in discussions and divulging your triumphs and tribulations, you naturally become an integral member of a dynamic, thriving network. These forums are treasure troves brimming with the collective wisdom of countless green thumbs, where you can delve into years of archived discussions or initiate a fresh thread about your latest horticultural puzzle. It's akin to having a virtual panel of gardening experts at your disposal.

The benefits of forging online gardening connections extend far beyond the convenience of virtual interaction. They present unparalleled access to diverse perspectives and expert insights, greatly enriching your comprehension of horticultural practices. You may stumble upon innovative techniques elucidated by someone cultivating plants in an entirely different climate or discover novel plant varieties thriving under similar conditions. Remarkably, these digital communities cultivate friendships that transcend the constraints of geographical boundaries. Envision exchanging seeds with an avid gardener situated oceans away or embarking on collaborative projects with someone whose acquaintance remains digital. These serendipitous connections undeniably enhance your gardening experience, continually reminding you that your endeavors form part of something infinitely grander: a global family of passionate plant lovers.

Numerous success stories underscore the profound impact of online gardening initiatives. Virtual garden tours offer the remarkable opportunity to explore breathtaking landscapes from the comfort of your couch. At the same time, engrossing webinars provide invaluable learning opportunities from esteemed experts without the need to venture from home. These events breathe life into gardens, rendering them accessible to anyone with an internet connection. Online plant swaps and seed exchanges catalyze platforms for sharing resources and knowledge, ensuring that unique and rare plant varieties continue to thrive globally. Such visionary projects succinctly illustrate the incredible potential of digital spaces to inspire innovation and foster collaboration amongst gardeners worldwide.

As we draw this chapter on gardening with community and

connection to a close, please take a moment to reflect on the profound manner in which these digital interactions broaden our horizons and deepen our profound appreciation for the fascinating world of plants. They remind us that although our gardens may be physically planted in our backyards, they are part of a far-reaching ecosystem comprised of shared knowledge and unwavering support. Whether cultivating plump tomatoes or tending to delicate, exotic orchids, always remember that somewhere lurks an individual ready and willing to proffer advice or revel in your jubilation.

Together, we shall unearth and explore myriad methods to nurture our botanical friends and our planet, ensuring that each unique garden flourishes with purpose and meticulous care. Ultimately, every plant we cultivate is a testament to our shared obligation as conscientious stewards of this breathtaking Earth, an endeavor best undertaken collectively for the betterment of all.

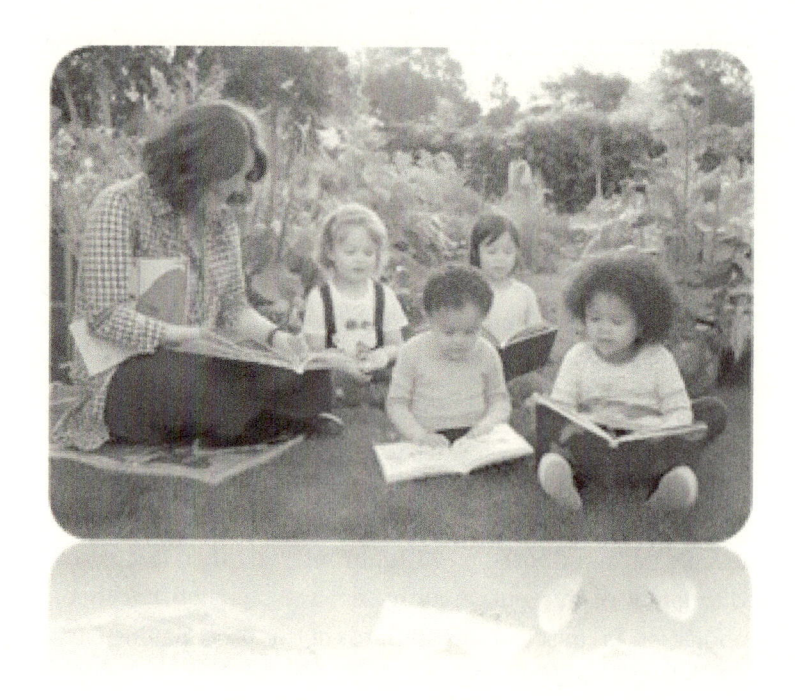

Storytime in the Garden: Engaging Children with Plant Tales

Once upon a time, in a garden not so far away, plants and people lived together in harmony. If this sounds like the beginning of a fairy tale, that's because it is, and rightly so! Storytelling possesses an enchanting way of capturing imaginations and imparting valuable lessons, particularly when it concerns captivating children with the wonders of gardening. Imagine this idyllic scene: you're leisurely seated under the dappled shade of a grand, old tree, surrounded by a small but eager audience of kids whose eyes are wide with anticipation.

CHAPTER 7

As you begin to weave a tale of magical gardens where flowers chatter and trees whisper secrets, suddenly, gardening isn't merely a task involving soil and seeds but an enthralling adventure just waiting to be unveiled.

Incorporating storytelling into gardening activities does more than transform learning about plants into an adventure; it introduces an epic quest filled with imagination and intrigue. Picture narrating the journey of a courageous tiny seed whose greatest dream is to grow into a magnificent towering tree. It bravely faces challenges like harsh droughts and pesky, hungry squirrels and learns to thrive despite obstacles. Fairy tales with enchanted gardens whisk children away to realms where the impossible becomes possible, motivating them to see their backyards as places brimming with potential and wonder. Fables revolving around plant life cycles and ecosystems unfold crucial concepts, making them both relatable and remarkable. Through such enchanting storytelling, children acquaint themselves with the wonders of the natural world and cultivate empathy for the living beings that inhabit it, fostering a lifelong appreciation for the environment.

But why limit the experience to just verbal storytelling? Transform it into an interactive journey! Encourage kids to embody roles from these tales, symbolically taking part in their own garden quests. Perhaps they'll take on the esteemed role of the sun, generously bestowing warmth upon budding seedlings, or energetically pretend to be a diligent bee buzzing from flower to flower, ensuring pollination. Acting out these captivating tales aids in fixing their understanding of plant growth stages and the myriad roles various elements play in sustaining the ecosystem. This hands-on, imaginative approach renders the learning process absorbingly fun and ignites children's creativity, critical thinking, and problem-solving skills.

Creating themed story gardens elevates this concept to an entirely new level. Imagine a "Jack and the Beanstalk" garden featuring climbing beans that ambitiously reach for the clouds or an "Enchanted Forest," adorned with twinkling fairy lights and charming decorations inviting exploration. These themed landscapes welcome children into a narrative wonderland where they can engage with nature imaginatively. In tending these themed gardens and witnessing firsthand the magical transformation plants undergo, they become integral characters in the ongoing story they help unfold.

The educational value of plant narratives is vast and profound. These stories serve as a springboard to teaching scientific principles in a playful, engaging manner. For example, stories detailing plant anatomy can help children retain the function of each part—roots that sip nourishing water, leaves that bask in the sunlight, and flowers that entice pollinators with their vibrant allure. Through storytelling, complex ideas morph into titillating and tangible knowledge, sparking curiosity and fostering an unquenchable thirst for further understanding. Moreover, stories can gently introduce environmental conservation topics, seamlessly teaching the critical importance of sustaining our planet's health through rich narratives showcasing the charm of nature's interconnected systems.

Visual Element: Story Garden Design Inspiration Chart

CHAPTER 7

- **Jack and the Beanstalk Garden:** Integrate tall bean poles with informative signage that narrates Jack's legendary tale, drawing kids into the adventure.
- **Enchanted Forest:** Sprinkle magical fairy lights and decorative, whimsical mushrooms to create an otherworldly, dreamlike ambiance.
- **Rainbow Garden:** Cultivate flowers in vivid color blocks, each representing different story themes and invoking vibrant imagery.
- **Butterfly Haven:** Develop winding pathways with stepping stones leading towards plants that magnetize butterflies, creating a living storybook.

Storytelling in the garden is far from a child's delight alone; it offers adults the delightful escapade of reconnecting with their inner child. It serves as a charming reminder that gardening transcends mere seed planting; it's about fostering growth, discovering captivating new worlds, and sharing life's enchanting experiences with others. By sowing the seeds of wonder through story-rich experiences, we nurture future generations to value and protect the natural world's beauty and intricate complexity.

Storytelling metamorphoses gardens into boundless classrooms, where every leaf harbors a lesson, and each bloom conceals a secret. Whether you're spinning tales of ancient plant myths or fashioning new adventures with your little ones, remember that each story enriches the garden's multifaceted experience. Perhaps one day, some of these children will evolve into passionate gardeners themselves, excitedly sharing the tales they've cherished to spark inspiration for yet another blossoming generation of green thumbs.

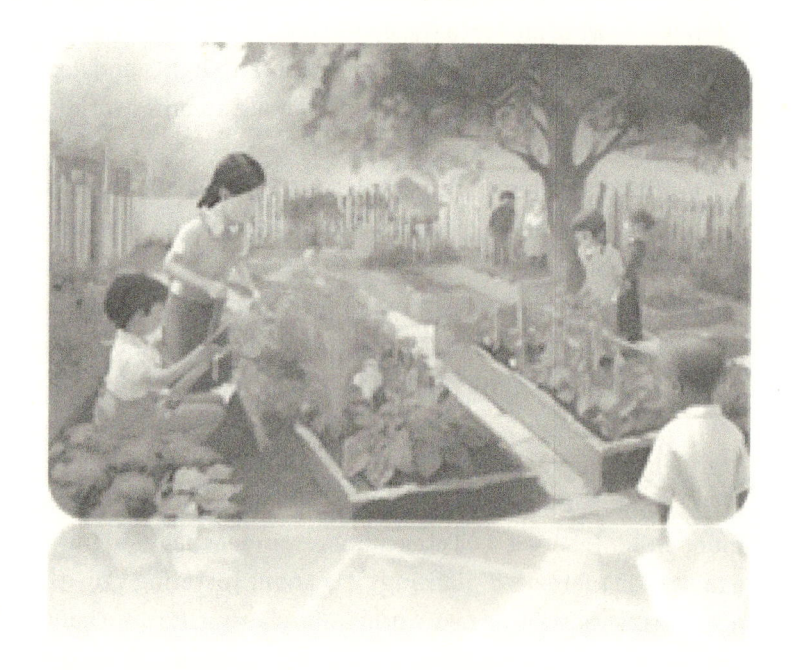

The Formative Influence of School Gardens

Imagine stepping into a world where the traditional confines of a classroom dissolve into nature's vibrant colors and textures. School gardens are not only a place for budding horticulturists but are also sacred grounds that foster young minds to think creatively and divergently. By swapping textbooks for trowels, students gain a multifaceted educational experience that reaches far beyond conventional boundaries. This setting becomes an invaluable educational asset, turning theoretical knowledge into tangible, hands-on exploration. Such environments do more than teach; they inspire and motivate, enabling students to cultivate plants and their burgeoning imaginations and understanding of the world.

Establishing these verdant learning environments involves more than just physical transformations; it requires the soulful investment of community members. Creating and nurturing these garden spaces becomes a shared journey—an expression of community spirit and a celebration of learning. Imagine "Garden Days," where laughter and the spirit of cooperation echo alongside the sounds of spades hitting the earth. Each family and volunteer brings unique capabilities to the mosaic of activities, building not just physical garden spaces but also memories and partnerships that can outlast the growing seasons.

Educational Integration and Beyond

Teachers, as facilitators of knowledge, play a decisive role in weaving garden activities into the educational fabric. The potential is limitless. Envision mathematics intertwined with nature, as students can calculate the growth rate of their plantings or prepare charts categorizing the various species in their plots. History classes can explore climate patterns, ancient irrigation techniques, and historical uses of different plants. A hands-on science curriculum comes alive amid rows of vegetables, with lessons in photosynthesis, soil health, and the energy cycles as children witness real-life biology unfold before their eyes. These evolving gardens become dynamic classrooms in themselves, offering ever-changing landscapes for the growth of both flora and intellect.

Developing gardens that complement school settings requires ingenuity and understanding students' needs. With their ease of use and defined boundaries, the use of raised beds turns abstract concepts into visible, touchable education modules. Sensory gardens further enhance the learning experience, offering a rich palette of experiences that seduce the senses. Imagine walking through a garden where the gentle rustle of leaves combines with the earthy fragrance of rosemary or where touching the soft fuzziness of sage leaves sparks curiosity, making the learning both memorable and multisensory. These are experiences that students can smell, feel, and even savor, making education immersive and holistic.

Practical Benefits and Lifelong Lessons

Beyond academics, school gardens serve as thriving personal and team development laboratories. In these shared spaces, students master the art of negotiation and cooperation as they work towards a collective vision. Projects like creating compost piles or designing a small ecosystem from local flora become lessons in collaboration, persistence, and patience. Moreover, these gardens are precursors to healthier living, where students, by tending their crops, become more adventurous in their culinary explorations. They learn to savor the crispness of freshly picked lettuce or the sweetness of garden-grown berries, a firsthand experience that initiates enduring healthy eating habits.

Exploring examples of successful school gardens unveils inspiring narratives of student empowerment and innovative projects. Imagine the camaraderie and excitement as students harness creativity to form garden clubs, leading initiatives with pride and responsibility. They become stewards of their patches, learning when to plant, nurture, and harvest, along with the associated risks and rewards, key life skills in responsibility and decision-making. Novel projects like crafting garden art from recycled objects or using rain barrels for irrigation help students apply critical thinking and sustainable practices in everyday contexts.

Building Community and Heritage

The advantages of school gardens ripple into the broader community, fostering idiosyncratic collaborations. Local businesses might contribute with garden materials or share water-saving technologies, embedding a sense of local pride and investment. Families, too, bring diverse knowledge bases, offering heirloom seeds and ancestral gardening wisdom to enrich garden education. This web of community participation and support weaves a tapestry of collective ownership that bolsters both the gardens' and the students' resilience.

School garden exploration traverses scientific phenomena, artistic creation, and historical insights through hands-on approaches, cultivating inquisitiveness about our surroundings while nurturing environmental respect. As students diligently attend to their horticultural duties, they join a cycle much larger than themselves, learning about ecosystems, organic growth, and the principles of sustainability, which all lay a robust groundwork for lifelong environmental stewardship.

With every planted seed, students engage in a quest of discovery, cultivating skills ranging from empathy to environmental consciousness that transcends the classroom. Here, in these fertile grounds, creativity blossoms, cooperation blooms, and connections flourish, nurturing crops and the next generation of earth-conscious citizens. School gardens thus signify a holistic educational approach that embarks on an enduring quest to sow seeds of wisdom, ecological respect, and communal harmony.

Garden Journals: Documenting Your Green Journey

Imagine standing in your garden, the morning sun casting a golden glow over dewy leaves, and you're holding a cup of coffee in one hand and a notebook in the other. This is the magic of garden journaling. It's your personal scrapbook of nature's marvels, recording everything from the first sprout to the final harvest. Think of it as your garden's biography, tracking growth, celebrating victories, and tackling challenges. With each entry, you become more in tune with your garden's rhythm. You discover which plants thrive, struggle, and surprise you by flourishing against all odds. A journal documents these nuances, turning fleeting moments into treasured memories.

Starting a garden journal is like picking out a new pair of shoes; they must fit your style. Some folks swear by the tactile joy of traditional paper journals, where you can feel the texture of each page and jot down notes with a favorite pen. Others embrace the convenience of digital journals, which offer easy organization and the ability to include photos with a quick tap. Whichever route you choose, the key is consistency. Regular entries create a comprehensive timeline of your garden's evolu-

CHAPTER 7

tion. Add sketches of your layout plans or photos capturing that moment when the sunflowers bloomed. These visual elements breathe life into your notes, providing context and sparking memories later on.

Now, let's talk about adding some flair. Your journal doesn't have to be all business; inject some fun and creativity into it! Try using color-coded entries for different plant species so you can easily flip through to find last year's tomato triumphs or this season's herb experiments. Pressed flowers and leaves make charming keepsakes, preserving your garden's beauty even in the dead of winter. These mementos add a tactile element that transforms your journal from mere record-keeping to a sensory experience. You'll find yourself flipping through past pages not just for information but for the sheer joy of reminiscing.

Journaling isn't just about recording what's happened; it's also about learning and growing as a gardener. As you document each season's experiments and outcomes, patterns begin to emerge. You may notice that peppers always do better with a bit of afternoon shade or that your roses bloom more after a spring rain. These insights inform future decisions, helping you refine your techniques and approach with each passing year. Your journal becomes a guidebook tailored to your specific garden's quirks and needs.

Imagine this: last summer, you tried planting marigolds alongside your tomatoes as a natural pest deterrent. You carefully noted the results in your journal: fewer aphids and healthier tomatoes! Next year, when planning your garden layout, you'll revisit those notes and replicate what worked well. This trial, reflection, and adjustment process propels you toward gardening success.

Interactive Element: Garden Journaling Checklist

- **Choose Your Format:** Decide between digital or traditional paper journals based on preference.
- **Include Visuals:** Incorporate photos, sketches, or pressed flowers for added context.
- **Color Code Entries:** Use different colors for various plant species or stages.
- **Regular Updates:** Set aside time weekly to record observations and changes.
- **Reflect on Results:** Review past entries to identify patterns and successes.

By documenting your gardening adventures, you create a living archive that enriches both your gardening journey and personal growth. This practice isn't just for seasoned gardeners; beginners can benefit immensely, too. Whether you're noting which seeds germinate fastest or capturing the joy of tasting your first homegrown strawberry, each entry builds confidence in your growing skills.

A garden journal acts as a bridge between seasons, linking past experiences to future aspirations. It keeps your gardening dreams alive through winter's chill and fuels spring-awakening anticipation. Over time, you'll discover that this simple habit enhances your gardening prowess and deepens your connection with nature's cycles. Through journaling, you'll cultivate plants, mindfulness, and appreciation for life's small wonders.

So grab that notebook or open that app; it's time to capture the essence of your green paradise!

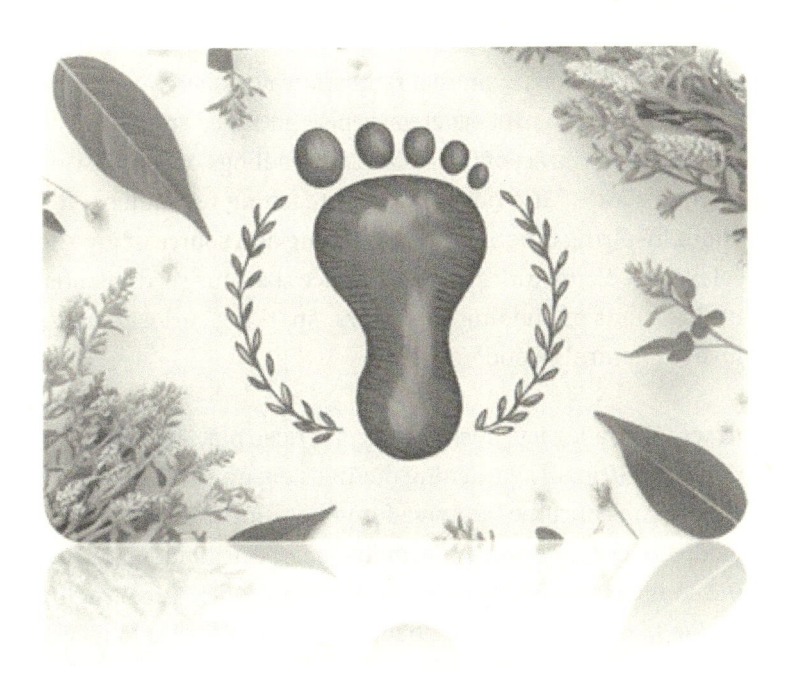

The Legacy of Gardening: Leaving a Green Footprint

Imagine standing in your garden, surrounded by the fruits of your labor, knowing that the knowledge you've gained is a treasure trove waiting to be shared. Passing on gardening wisdom is more than a kindness; it's a gift to future generations.

Consider penning your thoughts in a gardening guide or recipe book, turning your experiences into stories others can follow. Your book could include everything from soil tips to the perfect salsa recipe made from homegrown tomatoes. Imagine the joy you'd feel knowing someone miles away is savoring a dish inspired by your wisdom.

Hosting workshops is another fantastic way to share your expertise. Picture a group of eager gardeners gathered around as you demonstrate the art of transplanting seedlings or composting kitchen scraps. It's not just about teaching techniques; it's about inspiring others to see gardening as a source of joy and relaxation. Your stories and experiences become seeds planted in the minds of budding gardeners, sparking curiosity and a love for nature's wonders.

In weaving a legacy, sustainable practices play a crucial role. Using eco-friendly gardening methods ensures that our green spaces can continue to thrive for generations. By promoting biodiversity, we're protecting individual species and supporting the complex web of life that sustains our planet. Encouraging native plants and creating habitats for pollinators like bees and butterflies are simple yet powerful actions. These practices allow our gardens to become vibrant ecosystems that contribute positively to the environment.

Conservation techniques can be easily implemented in personal gardens. Rainwater harvesting, for example, is an efficient way to conserve water while nourishing your plants. Composting kitchen waste reduces landfill contributions and enriches soil naturally. These small changes add up, leaving a lasting impact

CHAPTER 7

on both your garden and the planet. By embracing these sustainable habits, you set an example for others, encouraging them to consider their own ecological footprints.

Creating a family gardening tradition is another fantastic way to pass down your love for gardening. Establish annual family planting days where everyone gets their hands dirty together, from toddlers to grandparents. These events can be as simple or elaborate as you like, starting with planting a new tree each year or dedicating a plot for vegetables the whole family can tend to and harvest. Such traditions foster a sense of responsibility and connection to the earth, teaching younger generations the importance of nurturing both plants and relationships.

Sharing family gardening stories and heirloom seeds adds depth to these traditions. Imagine telling tales of how your great-grandfather grew prize-winning zucchinis or how your grandmother's roses were the talk of the town. These stories enrich the gardening experience, transforming it into more than just planting and harvesting. Heirloom seeds carry the essence of these tales, embodying family history and resilience. By saving and passing them down, you ensure that future generations can enjoy the same flavors and beauty that have delighted your family for years.

Throughout history, many individuals have left indelible marks through their gardening legacies. Community leaders who transformed neglected public spaces into lush gardens have inspired countless others. Their efforts create havens for local wildlife while offering sanctuary and beauty for human visitors. These green oases become gathering places for neighbors, sparking conversations and fostering community spirit.

Generational family farms are another testament to the enduring power of gardening legacies. These farms are often passed down through multiple generations, and they maintain traditional practices while adapting to modern challenges. They serve as living examples of how sustainable farming methods can thrive alongside technological advancements. By sharing their stories and techniques, these farmers inspire others to appreciate the value of preserving agricultural heritage.

In leaving a gardening legacy, you contribute to something greater than yourself, a network of knowledge, beauty, and sustainability that touches lives beyond your own garden gate. Each act of sharing, teaching, and conserving ripples outward, creating a greener world where future generations can flourish alongside the plants we cherish today.

Imagine your garden as a canvas where you paint with seeds and sprouts, each stroke telling a story of growth and resilience. It's a place where memories are made, lessons are learned, and young hands discover the magic of nurturing life from soil to bloom. As you cultivate this space, know that you're not just growing plants; you're sowing seeds of inspiration and knowledge that will take root in hearts and minds for years to come.

In this shared adventure, we find joy in watching others blossom alongside their gardens, knowing that our legacy will continue long after we've set down our trowels. It's about creating connections between ourselves, our gardens, and those

CHAPTER 7

who will follow in our footsteps, ensuring the love for all things green endures through every season of life.

Gardening isn't just about the plants; it's about the transformative journey you embark upon alongside them. Each tender sprout breaking through the soil, every vibrant bloom unfurling its petals, and the bountiful harvest that rewards your toil with fresh produce are landmarks of personal growth and accomplishment that deserve to be celebrated with joy and pride. Picture yourself hosting a delightful garden party as a celebratory occasion to mark these achievements. Invite friends and neighbors, each one providing the harmonious chorus that resonates with the vibrant life you have created in your garden. Arrange tables amidst the verdant rows of veggies and resplendent flowers, laden with sumptuous dishes crafted from your own lovingly grown produce. This is more than just a gathering; it is a tribute to your unwavering dedication and hard work. Revel in the success of those first tomatoes ripening with luscious perfection and the roses blooming with a breathtaking brilliance that exceeds all expectations. Commemorating these milestones with others deepens their significance and adds layers of meaning and shared happiness, transforming your triumphs into cherished, collective memories that linger in the warmth of fellowship.

Another profoundly rewarding way to encapsulate your garden's journey is by creating photo albums or scrapbooks. This documentation of progress, from the timid first seedling striving for light to the mighty boughs of a fully grown plant, serves as a reservoir of memories and a reflective tool that informs future gardening endeavors. This collection of images and notes enables you to trace your advancement over time, highlighting what strategies proved most effective. Craft pages filled with contrasting before-and-after photographs, delicately preserved flowers, and handwritten notes that poignantly express your journey. This scrapbook evolves into a testament to your evolution not just as a gardener but as an individual, capturing moments of victory and the insightful lessons learned from challenges faced along the way

As you pause to reflect on your garden's growth, consider the personal growth intertwined with it. Gardening isn't simply about cultivating plants; it cultivates you. It instills resilience and galvanizes problem-solving skills like few other pastimes can. When confronted with an army of aphids or the onset of unexpected frosts, you hone your ability to adapt, devising innovative strategies to ensure the garden continues to flourish regardless of adversity. These challenges act as a forge, building resilience and teaching you the art of perseverance and patience, preparing you to navigate challenges with grace in all areas of life. Alongside resilience, gardening fosters mindfulness. The rhythmic routine of planting, weeding, watering, and nurturing the green growing life provides a soothing, meditative solace from life's stresses, an oasis where the world's clamor recedes, leaving you cloaked in a comforting peace.

Gardening is a canvas for setting new ambitions and planning future undertakings. It's time to consider expanding your diligent care to a larger garden space or diving into the thrilling experimentation of planting new and unfamiliar varieties. Setting these goals projects a beacon of excitement onto your gardening path, driving you to discover new, uncharted territo-

CHAPTER 7

ries in the wondrous world of horticulture. Joining community gardening projects can multiply these joys, allowing you to lend your green thumb to more significant initiatives while reaping the wealth of knowledge provided by fellow gardeners. These projects are the fertile soil from which personal satisfaction, collaboration, and a sense of belonging within a community bonded by their shared passion for growing life spring forth.

Sharing the bounty of your gardening experiences is yet another wonderfully enriching aspect of this pursuit. An unparalleled joy is derived from connecting with others over the fruits (and veggies) of your labor. Offering your surplus produce or seeds to neighbors sparks delightful conversations filled with tips, stories, and culinary inspirations and knits the community tighter through these gifts of the earth. Participate in gardening forums and networks to exchange advice, stories, and encouragement, making your journey richer through these virtual camaraderie bonds

The joy of sharing transcends produce, extending into the realm of knowledge. Contributing to gardening forums and networks enhances the collective pool of wisdom from which everyone benefits. Whether imparting sage advice on efficient pest control or gleaning innovative techniques from fellow enthusiasts, these exchanges foster an inclusive, nurturing environment where all can flourish.

As we conclude this reflective chapter, remember that gardening embraces growth in every dimension. Celebrating milestones, reflecting on personal development, setting goals that push boundaries, and generously sharing experiences enrich the tapestry of your gardening adventure. Your garden is a living testament to dedication and devotion, a sanctuary where memories unfurl, and the seeds of dreams are planted and nurtured.

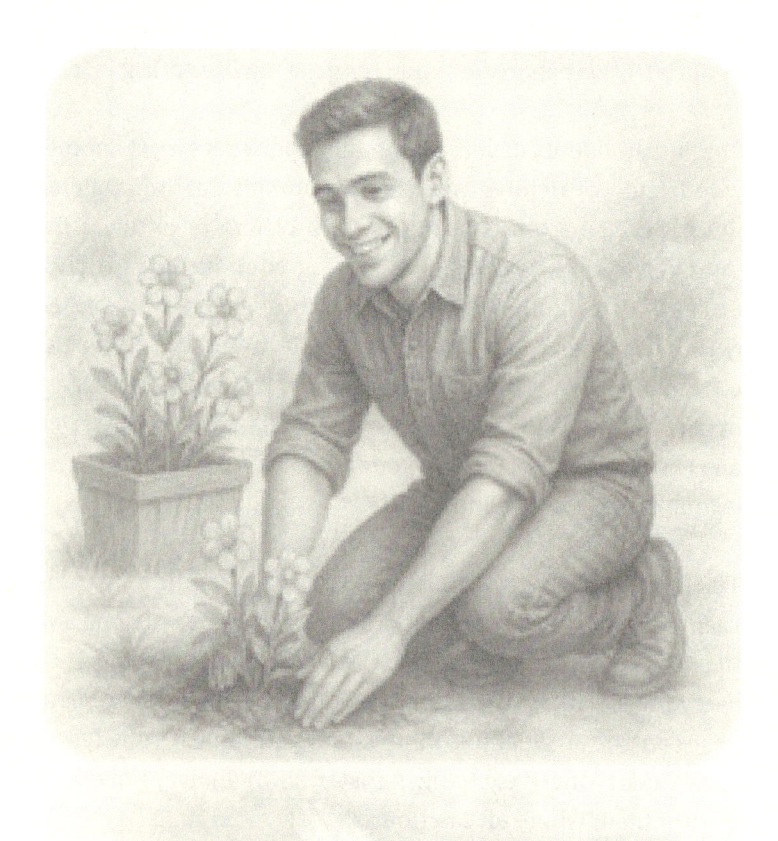

Chapter 8

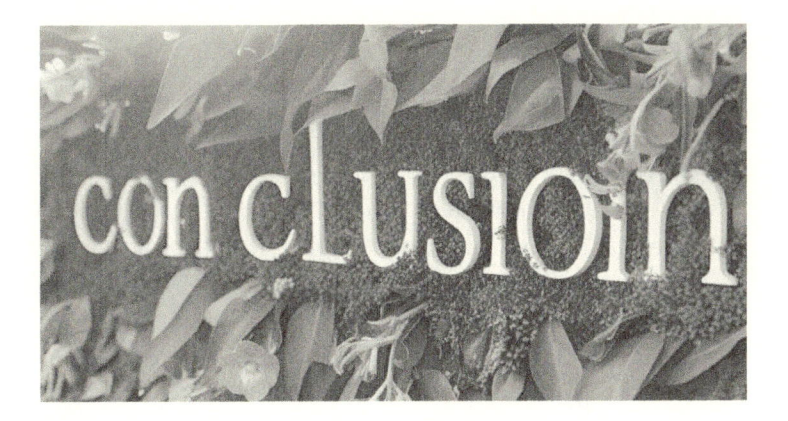

Conclusion

Well, here we are at the end of our journey through the lush, green world of gardening. It's been quite an adventure. From the moment you decided to pick up this book, you embarked on a path that intertwines with nature in the most rewarding ways. Whether cultivating vegetables, nurturing flowers, or simply enjoying the rustle of leaves in the breeze, gardening is a fulfilling pursuit connecting us with the natural world.

Gardening is more than just a hobby; it's a gateway to a healthier mind and body. Research shows that spending time in gardens can reduce stress, improve mood, and even boost physical health through light exercise. Your garden is a sanctuary, a place where you can escape the hustle and bustle and find peace among the plants. It's an educational pursuit, too, offering endless lessons about life, growth, and the importance of patience.

Throughout this book, we've covered many topics, haven't we? We've delved into the quirks of plant diversity, the magic of seeds, and the art of creating a pollinator paradise. You've learned about sustainable practices that benefit your garden and the planet. And let's not forget the fun projects and engaging activities that have brought a smile to your face along the way.

You've done more than just read; you've grown. Each page turned has been a step forward in your gardening journey, and I hope you've got soil under your nails to prove it. You've tackled projects, experimented with new techniques, and maybe even discovered a few surprises in your own backyard. Celebrate these achievements! Every sprout that breaks through the soil, every bloom that unfurls, is a testament to your dedication and curiosity.

Keep that curiosity alive. The gardening world is vast and full of wonders waiting to be discovered. Try new plants, explore different designs, and continue experimenting with sustainable

CHAPTER 8

methods. Gardening is a lifelong learning experience, and there's always something new to try. The more you explore, the more you'll understand the delicate balance of ecosystems and how you can contribute positively.

Now, here's a little nudge to take your passion beyond the garden gate. Share your experiences with others. Join a local gardening club or participate in plant swaps. Teach your neighbors and inspire future generations to dig into the dirt. Community engagement enriches your gardening experience and spreads the joy and benefits of gardening to others. Imagine the impact we can have when we all come together with a shared love for plants and nature!

Thank you for joining me on this green-thumb adventure. It's been a privilege to share these insights, tips, and stories with you. I hope this book has enriched both your life and your gardening practices. I'm grateful for your time and dedication.

Before we part ways, I'd love to hear from you. Your feedback and experiences are invaluable. They help create a dialogue that benefits us all. Feel free to share your successes, challenges, and favorite gardening mishaps. Connect with fellow enthusiasts and me so we can continue to grow together.

So, here's to you, the gardener, the dreamer, and the explorer. May your garden be ever bountiful, your heart full of joy, and your spirit forever curious until we meet again, happy gardening!

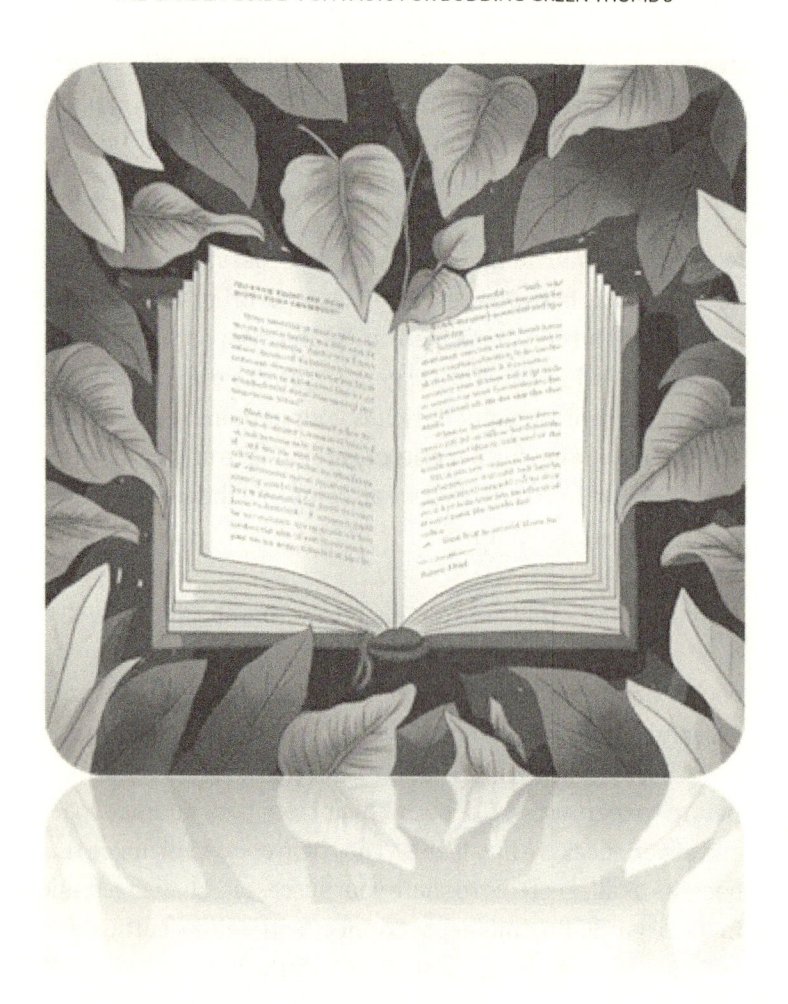

Book Review

If you enjoyed this book, please leave me a review. Your feedback will help me develop new garden books. Also, let me

CHAPTER 8

know if you enjoyed my book. Your review is critical to me and my upcoming series, which I am currently working on! Thank you for buying my book and reviewing its content.

Chapter 9

References

10 Mind-Blowing Facts about Plants. (2022, March 8). www.Click andgrow.com. Retrieved April 9, 2025, from https://www.click andgrow.com/blogs/news/10-mind-blowing-facts-about-pla nts

Gardening for health. (2018, June 18). https://pmc.ncbi.nlm.n ih.gov/articles/PMC6334070/

Hagen, L. (n.d.). *12 essential garden tools for the beginner*. www.gardendesign.com.

Debunking garden myths. (2023, July 5). www.extension.psu.edu. https://extension.psu.edu/debunking-garden-myth

Science Direct. (2024, December). *Phytoremediation: Harnessing plant power and innovative technologies for effective soil remediation*. www.sciencedirect.com. Retrieved April 9, 2025, from https://www.sciencedirect.com/science/article/pii/S266 7064X24002318

Wikipedia. (n.d.). *Tulip Mania*. en.wikipedia.org. Retrieved April 9, 2025, from https://en.wikipedia.org/wiki/Tulip_mani a

CHAPTER 9

Crop Trust. (n.d.). *Svalbard Global Seed Vault*. www.croptrust.org. Retrieved April 9, 2025, from https://www.croptrust.org/work/svalbard-global-seed-vault/

Yacon and malabar spinach - under the Solano sun. (n.d.). ucanr.edu. Retrieved April 9, 2025, from https://ucanr.edu/blogs/blogcore/postdetail.cfm?postnum=11404

Copeland, B. (2024, April 9). *How to Make a Miniature Fairy Garden*. Retrieved April 9, 2025, from https://www.marthastewart.com/how-to-make-a-fairy-garden-8628500

Ly, L. (n.d.). *The Beginner's No-Fail Guide to Starting Seeds Indoors*. Retrieved April 9, 2025, from https://gardenbetty.com/the-no-brainer-guide-to-starting-seeds-indoors/

Sorensen, D. (n.d.). *Plant Propagation - Cooperative Extension: Garden and Yard*. https://extension.umaine.edu. Retrieved April 9, 2025, from https://extension.umaine.edu/gardening/manual/propagation/plant-propagation/#:~:text=The%20major%20methods%20of%20asexual,plant%20parts%20from%20different%20varieties.

Koenig, M. (n.d.). *How to build a pollinator garden*. https://www.fws.gov. Retrieved April 9, 2025, from https://www.fws.gov/story/how-build-pollinator-garden

U.S. Department of Agriculture. (n.d.). *Benefits of organic Certification - Agricultural Marketing Service*. www.ams.usda.gov. Retrieved April 9, 2025, from https://www.ams.usda.gov/services/organic-certification/benefits#:~:text=Research%20shows%20that%20organic%20farming,Contribute%20to%20soil%20health

U.S, Department Of Energy. (n.d.). *Best Management Practice #5: Water-Efficient Irrigation*. www.energy.gov. Retrieved April 9, 2025, from https://www.energy.gov/femp/best-management-practice-5-water-efficient-irrigation

Iannotti, M. (2024, March 21). *What Is Mulch? How to Use 8 Types in Your Garden.* www.thespruce.com. Retrieved April 9, 2025, from https://www.thespruce.com/what-is-mulch-1402413

Landers, L. (n.d.). *How to use companion planting for garden pest control.* https://zerowastehomestead.com. Retrieved April 9, 2025, from https://zerowastehomestead.com/companion-gardening-guide-how-to-use-companion-planting-for-garden-pest-control/

Baldwin, D. L. (n.d.). *Succulent Container Design: Tips, Tricks & Inspiration.* https://debraleebaldwin.com. Retrieved April 9, 2025, from https://debraleebaldwin.com/succulent-container-design/

Chelsea Green Publishing. (n.d.). *Tips for the Square-Inch gardener: Vertical gardening.* www.chelseagreen.com. Retrieved April 9, 2025, from https://www.chelseagreen.com/2019/tips-for-the-square-inch-gardener-vertical-gardening-and-the-three-ts/#:~:text=There%20are%20three%20techniques%20involved,sunlight%20and%20space%20you%20have.

Midwest Living editors. (2023, March 23). *Garden art anyone can create.* www.midwestliving.com. Retrieved April 9, 2025, from https://www.midwestliving.com/garden/ideas/garden-art-anyone-can-create/

Sweetser, R. (2025, February 25). *Edible landscaping: selecting the right plants.* www.almanac.com. Retrieved April 9, 2025, from https://www.almanac.com/edible-landscaping-selecting-right-plants

University of Florida Extension. (n.d.). *Plant Diseases - Gardening solutions.* ufl.edu. Retrieved April 9, 2025, from https://gardeningsolutions.ifas.ufl.edu/care/pests-and-diseases/diseases/

Sowards, J. (2022, May 15). *Organic garden pest control.*

https://rootsandrefuge.com. Retrieved April 9, 2025, from https://rootsandrefuge.com/organic-garden-pest-control/

Hopper, B. (n.d.). *Soil Testing and Choices of Amendments - Extension Gardener.* https://extensiongardener.ces.ncsu.edu. Retrieved April 9, 2025, from https://extensiongardener.ces.ncsu.edu/2020/05/soil-testing-and-choices-of-amendments/

Screen Rants. (2023). *10 Gadgets & tools to make gardening easy in 2023.* https://screenrant.com.

Homestead Brooklyn. (2017, October 19). *How to organize a plant swap like a Pro!* https://homesteadbrooklyn.com. Retrieved April 9, 2025, from https://homesteadbrooklyn.com/all/2017/10/12/how-to-organize-a-plant-swap-like-a-pro

Public health benefits of community gardens. (2024, April 14). https://publichealth.tulane.edu. Retrieved April 9, 2025, from https://publichealth.tulane.edu/blog/benefits-of-community-gardens/

STATIONERS. (n.d.). *13 tips for throwing the perfect garden Party.* https://www.greenvelope.com. Retrieved April 9, 2025, from https://www.greenvelope.com/blog/tips-for-throwing-the-perfect-garden-party

Gonzalez, R. (2018, October 11). *10 online gardening communities you should join.* https://www.treehugger.com. Retrieved April 9, 2025, from https://www.treehugger.com/online-gardening-communities-you-should-join-4858500

Path of Learning. (n.d.). *12 outdoor storytelling techniques for kids that spark . . .* https://www.pathsoflearning.net. Retrieved April 9, 2025, from https://www.pathsoflearning.net/1976/outdoor-storytelling-techniques-for-kids/#:~:text=Plant%20Life%20Narratives&text=Feature%20stories%20about%20seed%20dispersal,growth%20patterns%20through%20engaging%20narratives

Plant a Seed See What Grows. (n.d.). *6 School garden examples to inspire your own.* https://seewhatgrows.org. Retrieved April 9, 2025, from https://seewhatgrows.org/6-school-garden-examples-to-inspire-your-own/

How to create a garden journal. (2023, January). https://piedmontmastergardeners.org. Retrieved April 9, 2025, from https://piedmontmastergardeners.org/article/how-to-create-a-garden-journal/

Better Homes and Gardens, Weir-Jimerson, K., & Hoppe Norgaard, C. (2025, January 2). *12 Sustainable Gardening Tips for an Eco-Friendly Yard.* https://www.bhg.com. Retrieved April 9, 2025, from https://www.bhg.com/gardening/yard/lawn-care/10-tips-for-sustainable-gardening/

Made in the USA
Coppell, TX
22 May 2025